D1423534

total home
workout

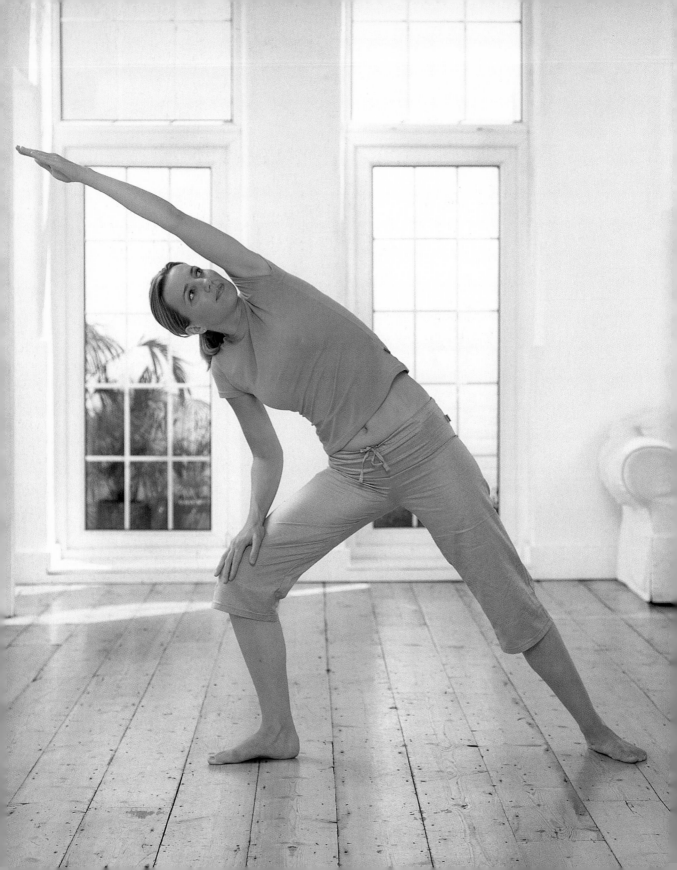

total home workout

A daily workout programme for total home fitness

Chrissie Gallagher-Mundy

First published in 2005 by
A&C Black Publishers Ltd
37 Soho Square, London W1D 3QZ
www.acblack.com

Conceived and produced by
Elwin Street Limited
79 St John Street
London EC1M 4NR
www.elwinstreet.com

A CIP catalogue record for this book is available
from the British Library.

Designer: Louise Leffler
Photographer: Mike Prior
Models: Lucy Baldwin and Karen Lanson
Clothes and equipment supplied by Bloch, Sweaty
Betty and Fitness Network

Printed in Singapore

While every effort has been made to ensure that the
content of this book is technically accurate and as
sound as possible, neither the author nor the publishers
can accept responsibility for any injury or loss sustained
as a result of use of this material.

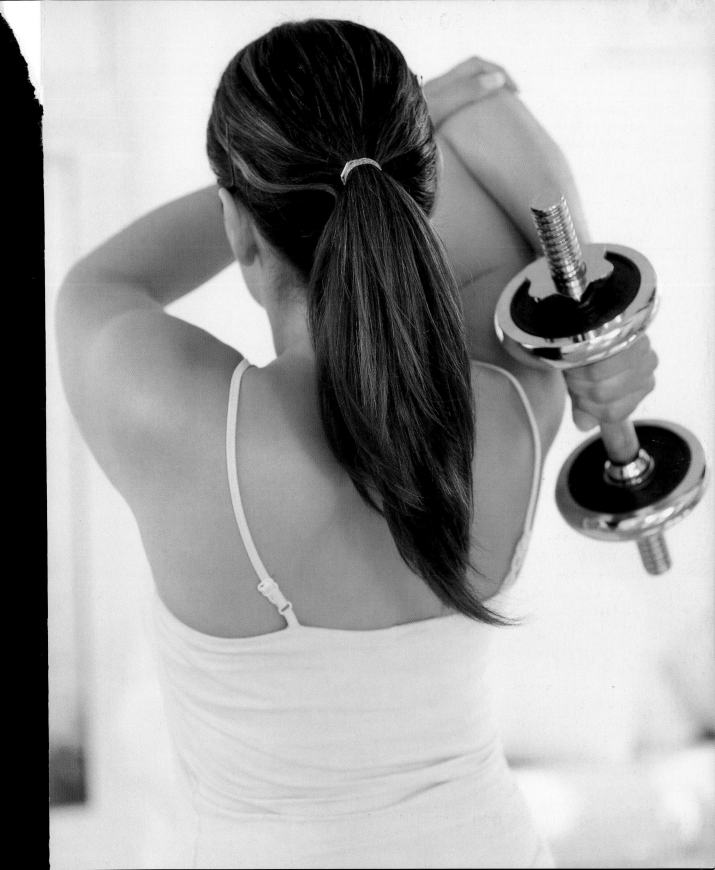

contents

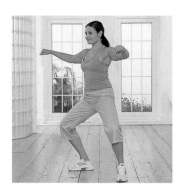 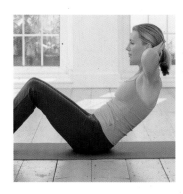 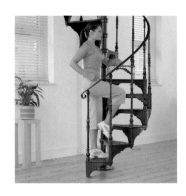

introduction

So you want the body of a Hollywood diva – Demi Moore's six-pack tummy, Madonna's sculpted shoulders or Beyonce's well-defined backside – but you don't have a celebrity income or an extra six hours a day? The good news is that you can get that look – and it's easier than you think. Even better, you don't need a fancy gym membership, a high-profile personal trainer or expensive machines that rival those in your local fitness centre. In fact, you don't even need to leave the house. The key to building a leaner, sexier and more toned body in record time starts with a few standard pieces of equipment (dumbbells, balls and bands), a designated space in your home and less than an hour a day for just three days a week. That's probably less time than you spend in your daily commute to work or standing in line for your morning latte.

Whether you're a gym rat looking to take a break from your weekly pump classes, a moderate exerciser who doesn't like the gym scene or a novice looking to start a routine in a non-threatening environment, this book will teach you everything you need to know about turning your humble abode into a super-effective body-shaping centre. You'll learn how to use your sofa to firm your bum and how your everyday dining-room chair can transform your triceps.

Not only that, the techniques listed here are the latest, greatest proven body sculptors taken from a variety of the hottest, most effective modalities such as yoga, Pilates, kick-boxing and more. In other words, you'll be learning the same powerful moves that get Hollywood actresses ready for the big screen and the red carpet. And because you know that the only way to truly lose weight is to burn more calories than you consume, combine these expert-approved moves with sensible eating habits and soon you'll have a fabulously toned body from head to toe.

Start by taking the quiz on page 13 to help you determine your fitness goals – a revved-up metabolism, a pumped-up cardiovascular system or pretzel-like flexibility. Then use that insight to create a personalised home-training programme that is specific to your needs. Once you build your routine, step-by-step instructions and photos ensure that the moves are simple to perform and easy to understand, which lessens your risk of injury and maximises your muscle-building results.

If this isn't enough to get off the sofa and ready to work out, consider this – people who work out don't just banish cellulite, blast fat and burn loads of calories, they also boost their mental and emotional wellbeing. Studies show that regular exercise combats depression, eases stress and helps you cope better with everyday anxiety, as well as bounce back from major life setbacks. The fitness makeover you find in these pages is guaranteed to give you rock-solid confidence, a healthy shot of self-esteem and an unshakable body image. Begin today and you'll join millions of other home exercisers on the fast-track to creating a super-fit body you love.

Stacy Baker
Fitness magazine

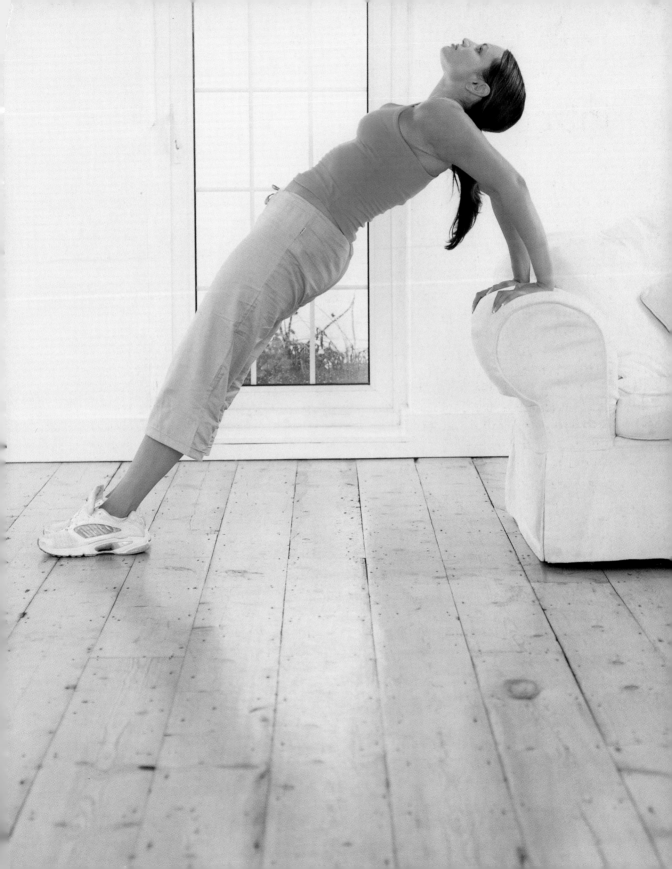

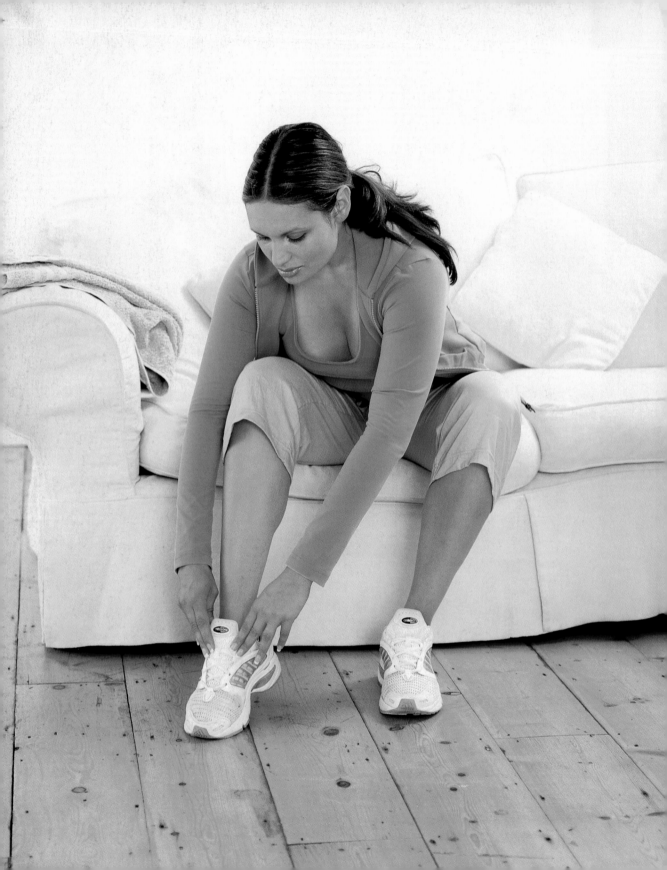

chapter 1

the joy of home training

Working out at home is a great way to form realistic, healthy habits and incorporate them into your weekly routine. The day-to-day lives of most women are extremely busy – the strains of juggling numerous demands at one time take their toll on our minds and bodies. Modern living, with its pollutants and stresses, can tire us, leaving us jaded and exhausted. Modern technology might make chores quicker, but because of such conveniences we perform less physical exercise. The joy of home training is that you don't need to go anywhere or spend lots of money in order to enhance your health and develop strength, fitness and tone.

The benefits of a home workout

Gyms and exercise studios can now be found in almost every town in every country – especially since obesity reached epidemic proportions in the West. When you consider the increase in the availability and consumption of rich foods, which are high in calories and gloriously tempting in their abundant variety, alongside our more sedentary lifestyles you can see why weight gain is a problem for many Western societies. Fitness centres are helping to raise awareness that moving around vigorously is beneficial not only in the prevention of weight gain but also in the prevention of diseases.

But gyms don't suit everyone. Even if you enjoy working out at the gym, no doubt there are times when you are hard-pressed to find the time to get there on a regular basis. A home workout routine that you can put into practice whenever you have a pocket of time is an invaluable tool for keeping fit.

If you are a gym-user or you enjoy going to dance or fitness classes, then having a personalised home workout will add to your regime. You can personally tailor the programme to cover elements of fitness that you wouldn't normally cover at the gym, or you can concentrate on specific elements of your training that need extra attention in order to move on to the next level.

If you are not someone who is motivated by gym training or workouts in a group situation then building a programme you can do in the comfort and privacy of your own home will inspire you to enjoy some regular exercise. You may even discover the joys of feeling fitter and more energetic than you ever have before.

The advantages of getting fit at home

▶ You don't have to make an appointment with anyone to exercise.

▶ You have more time to train because when you work out at home you don't waste time travelling there and back.

▶ You can perform your workout whenever you feel like it.

▶ You don't have to worry about the set time for a class or waiting for a piece of equipment to become available.

▶ You can feel comfortable and safe in your own home. This enhances your training time and means that you are inclined to train more often.

▶ You don't have to worry about what you're wearing (as long as it's safe) or who will see you – you will be in your own private gym.

▶ Fitness training at home doesn't need to be expensive or involve purchasing complicated pieces of equipment. Just a few inexpensive useful bits and pieces are all you need to get you on the road to fitness.

What is fitness?

First, let's consider the reasons you want to train. Complete the quiz opposite to gain some insight into your current fitness levels and what you regard as important to your fitness.

What do you want from a fitness programme?

1 Can you run for a bus a short distance down the road without feeling puffed?

2 Can you confidently climb a tall escalator without stopping for a rest?

3 Can you take three flights of stairs and immediately have a conversation with someone when you reach the top?

4 Do you feel physically exhausted at the end of most days?

5 Do you feel ready to leap up and get going first thing in the morning?

6 Do you feel mobile and agile?

7 Can you touch your toes when you are sitting with your legs straight out in front of you, on the floor?

8 Can you comfortably twist around in your chair to look at someone directly behind you?

9 Do you feel that you lack the strength to lift and carry heavy objects?

10 Do you worry that you have flabby-looking arms or a podgy stomach?

11 Do you wish you were thinner?

12 Does your posture need to be improved?

IF YOU ANSWERED **NO** TO ANY OF QUESTIONS 1 TO 4:

You need to work on your cardiovascular fitness. Cardio fitness concerns the wellbeing of the heart and lungs. The heart needs to be exercised and challenged to become more capable and strong. As you do this you also challenge the lungs. When these two body parts are fit, they work more efficiently, making it easier for you to run, walk up stairs and keep going throughout your day without feeling exhausted.

IF YOU ANSWERED **NO** TO ANY OF QUESTIONS 5 TO 8:

You are lacking flexibility. As you age, your body tightens up. Your movements become restricted if you maintain a sedentary lifestyle. The less you stretch, turn and twist, the less your muscles are prepared for it. This can result in stiffness and soreness when you do attempt to do something out of the ordinary and can even lead to injury when you overexert yourself. Flexibility training will ensure you maintain an ability to move comfortably in all directions.

IF YOU ANSWERED **YES** TO ANY OF QUESTIONS 9 TO 12:

You need to concentrate on muscle enhancement. This means putting your muscles under stress so that they will become stronger, more capable and more defined in shape. Strong, lean muscles burn more calories, ensure safe movement and keep the alignment of the body in place. As your body shape changes, you will shed inches, rather than mass.

How the body works

It is likely that when you did the quiz on the previous page there were elements in each section on which you felt you needed to improve. This is true for most of us. The word 'fitness' really just describes an all-round feeling of knowing you are physically capable of doing anything you feel like doing. When you say you want to feel 'fit', what you are probably describing is that feeling you had when you were a child: the liberating feeling of not worrying about your body and being able to run, jump, leap and bend without discomfort or restriction. When you are fit you feel capable, happy and full of confidence. You feel good and look good too.

Fitness enhances your mental facilities as well. When you concentrate on working out you enjoy a release of your usual thought patterns to do with work, relationships, money and other issues that you are dwelling on. As you focus on your physical body, your mind shifts into a different gear and you begin to relax – tuning in more to your subconscious and your deeper feelings. This means that exercise can really help you to deal with stress and worries and lift your spirits in very tangible ways.

The key to getting and feeling fit is to make sure that your home workout is a total body workout, covering a warm-up, cardio exercise and spot muscle training as well as cool-down, so that nothing is overlooked or neglected. Each main muscle group should feel challenged and extended by the end of a workout. This will keep your body in its most capable state. You will be free from injury, discomfort and ready for action.

This book provides you with the information you need to put all these key elements effectively and safely into your home workout sessions.

What elements should a home fitness programme include?

▶ Warm-up: this readies each major muscle group for work and prepares the mind to concentrate on the activity to come.

▶ Cardiovascular exercise: this challenges your heart and lungs and increases their capacity for work. This type of exercise includes brisk walking, jogging, jumping, skipping, running, hopping, stepping and rebounding. Another name for this exercise is 'aerobic' exercise.

▶ Strengthening work: this lengthens your muscle fibres. If you incorporate strengthening work into your lifestyle, you will look more toned and you will be more capable of lifting, pushing and pulling at a higher level of effectiveness.

▶ Flexibility work: this keeps your muscles limber, maintains a good range of movement and allows you to twist, turn and stretch without discomfort.

▶ Co-ordination work: this challenges your 'muscle memory', or the ability of your mind and body to process a series of movements. This type of exercise focuses your mind and helps your body move smoothly and elegantly.

▶ Balance work: this perfects your posture, helping to keep your body injury-free and looking good.

▶ Relaxation: focused breathing and other relaxation techniques not only ensure adequate intake of oxygen but also calm the mind and soothe the body.

Anatomy check-up

Before you start putting together your home workout programme, you may need to refresh your memory about the basic structures of the body, so that you know why and how to target each region. Principally, these are the heart and lungs and the main large muscles of the body. Take a look at page 16 for a quick ID guide to the target muscles.

Remember, muscles work by contraction, so if you want to tone a particular muscle group you need to contract it, preferably against resistance, to make it work hard and increase strength.

Setting up your home gym

You don't need to build a whole new room or clear out your dining room for your great new workout regime. If you do have a room you can devote to it, all the better; however, most of us don't have that luxury. Consider using the corner of your bedroom or any spare space in your living room for exercise. Wherever you choose to exercise, all you need is a little space and a calm, positive atmosphere conducive to focusing your mind on your fitness and wellbeing.

Check the basics

▶ Make sure your room has a minimum of 4 square metres of empty floor space. This might involve you moving some furniture around or out of the room or pushing the bed to one side. Ideally, this is easily done so you don't have to do a great deal of rearranging every time you attempt to work out.

▶ Open the window – you'll need ventilation once you start sweating.

▶ Check the floor surface. Carpet is fine for working out. It provides a soft surface to lie on and support for the spine. If you have wooden floors you might need to invest in an exercise or yoga mat for comfort when performing floor moves. If you have a rug on the floor be extra careful. If it does not rest on a really tough gripping underlay there is the risk that you might slip and fall. You might need to be prepared to roll it up each time you work out or even to leave it to one side or move it elsewhere for the foreseeable future.

▶ Don't worry if there are chairs, sofas and beds in the room. All these objects may come in useful during your workout. Cushions, throws and even belts or dressing-gown ties can all be used in your fitness programme. When you read the equipment checklist over the page, look around and be inventive. Also try to place a mirror in a position where you can see your full body. This will help you check your body alignment as you work.

▶ Have you got a radio or small stereo in this room? Music will help you keep working when the going gets tough.

▶ A noticeboard on the wall is a great idea. As you define your goals and types of workout, pin them up here. It will be easy to see when you are working out and you can refer to them constantly. This is a great motivator.

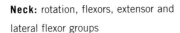

Key muscle groups of the body

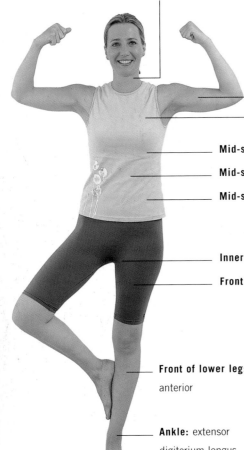

Neck: rotation, flexors, extensor and lateral flexor groups

Front of upper arm: biceps

Chest: pectoralis major

Mid-section: transverse

Mid-section: rectus abdominus

Mid-section: external and internal oblique

Inner thigh: adductors

Front of thigh: quadriceps

Front of lower leg: tibialis anterior

Ankle: extensor digitorium longus, extensor hallucis longus and peroneus tertius

Back of upper arm: triceps

Shoulders: trapezius, deltoids

Back: terus major, latissimus dorsi

Mid-section: abdominals

Lower back: erector group

Buttocks: gluteus maximus

Back and sides of thigh: iliotibial tract

Back of thigh: hamstrings

Back of lower leg: calf

Ankle: Achilles tendon

Professional equipment

There are some pieces of professional gym equipment that you may want to invest in to get the best out of your home workout. You might have some of these already or there might be some items around your home that will work as a substitute. Most of this equipment is inexpensive, easy to store and can be purchased from sports shops and department stores.

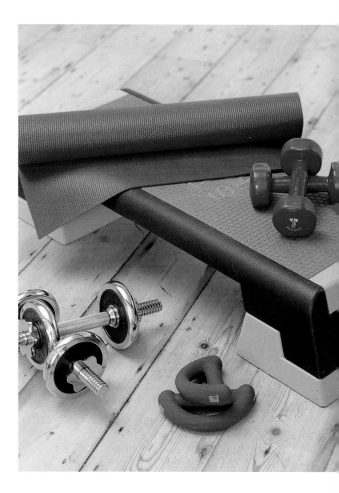

▶ A good pair of dumbbells is invaluable for muscle toning, so consider getting hold of a pair. The best types to buy are the ones that allow you to change the weights on the end by screwing off the collars. This allows you to increase and decrease the weight accordingly for each exercise you perform – and also to up the resistance as you get stronger. Each muscle group will be able to bear a different-sized load. These weights enable you to make the appropriate weight change when you move from one exercise to another.

▶ Yoga blocks are a good idea for some of the yoga moves. Thick books could be used as a substitute, but if you can find a yoga supplier, invest in two blocks for your training.

▶ Bands are great tools for toning your body, and a must for many Pilates-based moves.

▶ If you don't have a staircase in your house, or nearby outdoors, you may want to invest in a portable step to do some of the cardiovascular work. These can easily be stacked against a wall or slipped under a bed when not in use.

Getting started

What to wear

Now that you have your equipment and space organised, think about what to wear. Sports clothing that is made from breathable, supple fabrics and allows sweat to evaporate is ideal. However, any clothing that you find comfortable, conforms to your body and doesn't hinder movement will do fine.

▶ Make sure you have a good pair of trainers. Once you are training regularly and putting your shoes though their paces, you will need to replace them every six months. This ensures that your ankles and feet get optimal support and will go some way to avoid stress injuries.

▶ Wear layers of clothing. After the warm-up phase, you can peel off the layers. At the end of the workout you can then drape a layer back on to keep you warm during the final stages of your routine as you warm down.

▶ When doing some of the yoga and other floor work, you may want to work in bare feet. Working like this is a good way to exercise the feet and develop balance.

▶ If you have long hair or a hairstyle where your hair can get in your face, tie it back or use a head-band to keep it out of the way. You want to be as comfortable as possible with the minimum of distractions while you work out.

When should I train?

The time you have to train very much depends on your schedule, but bear in mind the following important points.

It is generally true that to notice improvement in exercise, you need to repeat it three times a week for at least six weeks. At this level of training you will notice significant fitness gains and changes in the shape of your body. You may need to sit down and think about your goals so that you can build a workout programme that works towards them (see chapter 2).

If your main goal is weight loss or weight main-tenance, building muscle tone and cardiovascular exercise are key. To see results, this should be done at least three times per week.

Most people find working out in the morning means the workout actually gets done more often than if they plan it later in the day. Could you possibly get out of bed an hour earlier to fit in your workout? The feeling of achievement you'll have for the rest of the day will make the early start worth it. You are also likely to feel more energetic and invig-orated for the rest of the day.

Make sure you train when you have enough food inside you. It's no good planning to work out at lunch time if this leaves you no time to eat either before or after. If it is not first thing in the morning, try to eat well before you plan to work out, perhaps an hour and a half before, and plan to eat again within two hours of your workout.

TRAINING TIP
Remember: it takes 30 days to form a habit.

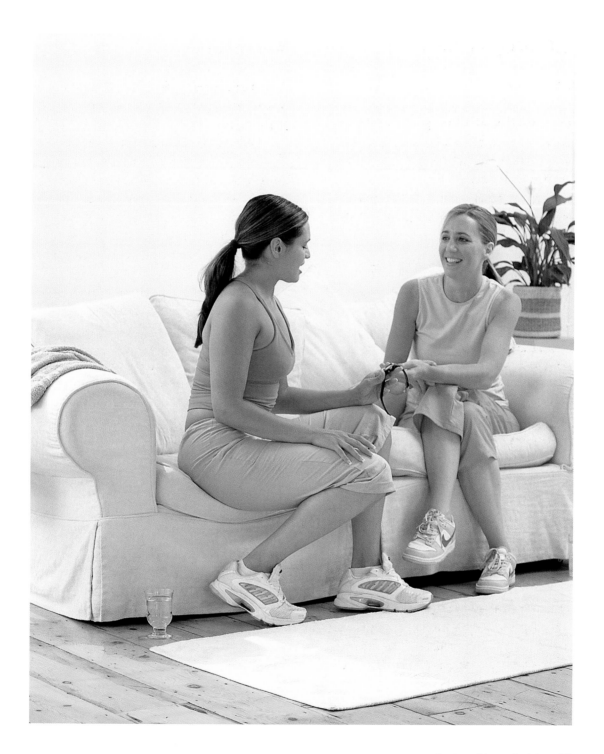

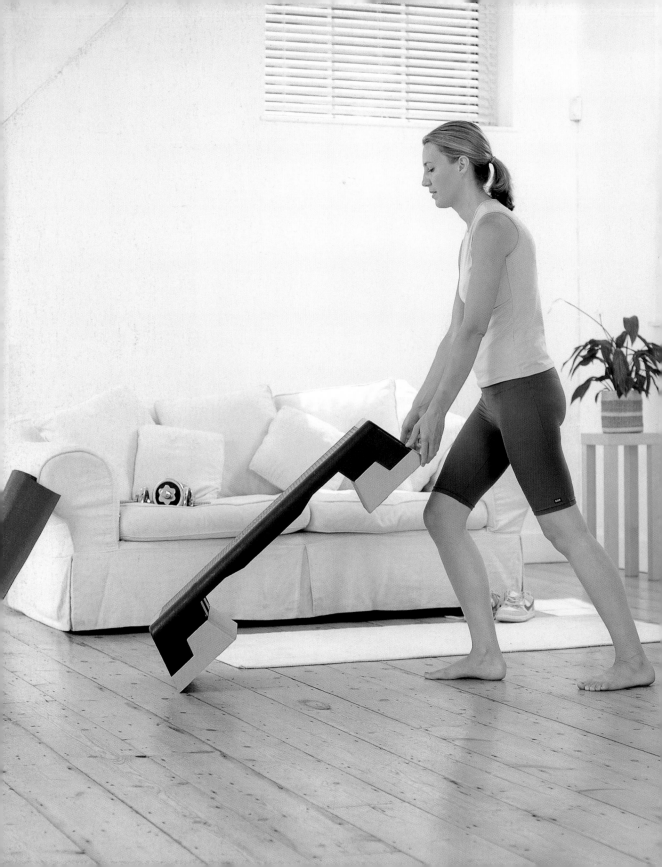

chapter 2

building your home workout

The type of workout you put together can vary. You don't have to stick with one particular option: the beauty of a home workout is that you can experiment and try all kinds of different things to keep you motivated and enthusiastic. Home workouts are more flexible than going to the gym or sitting on a piece of exercise equipment because you can alter them to suit your mood. If you are feeling a little under the weather, don't avoid exercising, simply choose a routine that seems a little gentler from your portfolio of workouts. If you're feeling really energetic, you can choose to do a more fast-paced workout than usual.

Your goals

In order to think what your home workout should consist of, your need to consider your fitness goals – what you would specifically like to achieve. The questions below offer some help in identifying these.

What are your personal exercise goals?

Reading down each column, place a 1, 2 or 3 beneath each quality to rank which is most important to you of these sets of qualities, where 3 is most important and 1 is least important.

WEIGHT LOSS	BEING THIN	LOSING INCHES	ALL-OVER WORK NEEDED	**Total score row A**
WEIGHT CONTROL	LOOKING ATHLETIC	FIRMING MUSCLES	TONING STOMACH AND ARMS	**Total score row B**
EASE OF MOVEMENT	BEING FLEXIBLE	ELONGATING MUSCLES	LOOSENING TIGHT BACK/HAMSTRINGS	**Total score row C**

Now you have completed this, add up your scores across the table to get a number value for rows A, B and C.

IF **A** WAS YOUR HIGHEST SCORE
This indicates your main focus is weight loss. If this is your key motivator then that's fine, you just have to make sure you have a plan for that. First you need to watch what you eat – a healthy diet is vital – and then you need to train every other day for at least 60 minutes.
Total time devoted to exercise per week:
4 hours

IF **B** WAS YOUR HIGHEST SCORE
This indicates your main focus is muscle toning. Your home workout can be simpler and less intense than a focus on weight loss. Training for 30 minutes every day will get you the body you want.
Total time devoted to exercise per week:
3 hours 30 minutes

IF **C** WAS YOUR HIGHEST SCORE
This indicates your main focus is mobility to keep supple and flexible. To achieve this you need to stretch regularly, training for 20 minutes every day.
Total time devoted to exercise per week:
2 hours 20 minutes

Committing yourself to fitness training

Now that you have a clear idea of your goals and the type of approach to exercise you may want to take, you can start thinking about where you will find the time to fit your home workout into your lifestyle. Use the chart below to make a commitment to yourself. It is commitment to regular exercise that will make the difference to your body. Deciding the kind of workout you need is important but doing the actual training is even more important. Photocopy and pin up this chart for the first few weeks of your training. It will remind you of the appointments you have made with yourself to exercise. Once you have been successful in this for a few weeks, you will find the regime becomes easier to stick to. You will also be encouraged as you see results.

Your time chart

Block out time in your weekly schedule that you honestly feel you can keep free for exercise. Bear in mind how many hours you need to exercise each week depending on your goals. Use the chart to plot blocks of time that you can fit into your day to make up the total hours required for the week. Keep in mind that 10 minutes isn't too short a period of time to schedule in; the 'corners of your day' can be used fruitfully to tone and shape your body.

	MON	TUE	WED	THUR	FRI	SAT	SUN	TOTAL TIME THIS WEEK
Morning								
Lunchtime								
Afternoon								
Evening								

Now you are ready for the final stage of the building blocks process. You just need to decide the real content of each of your workout blocks. On the following pages you will find a description of the various workouts that you can start to pick and choose from to build your first few weeks, then you can use the templates at the end of this chapter to draw up your final plans.

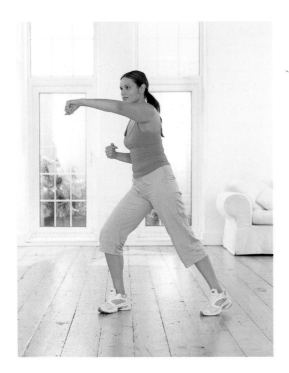

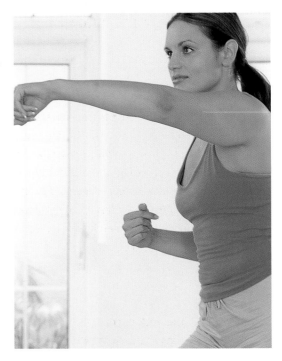

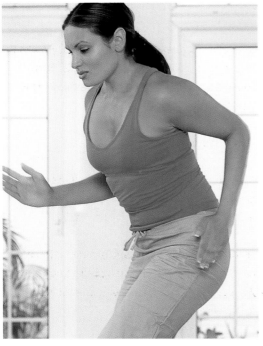

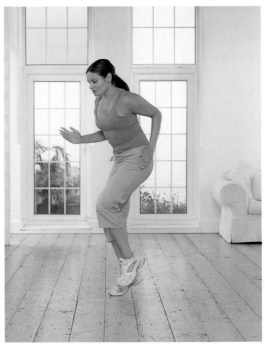

Your cardiovascular options

There are many different ways to work your cardio-vascular system. Any exercise that tends to use the large muscles of the body in a rhythmic motion will work this system. As you move consistently, the demand for oxygen increases and therefore so does the rate of breathing. The oxygen is then utilised in the energy-release process, facilitating a breakdown of fats for more energy. These are the cardiovascular activities included in this book.

Aerobics

Aerobics is really just another name for cardiovascular exercise but has come to mean dance-type moves strung together to music. In the pages that follow you will find numerous ideas for aerobic exercise, which you can put together to form a cardio routine. Put on some upbeat music of your choice and try first one move and then the next to form a continuous flow of movement. Don't get inhibited – it's all about having a go and keeping on going.

Walking

Walking is a great exercise that can everyone can enjoy. Just because anybody can do it, however, doesn't mean to say it has to be easy! Once you get into walking you can really start to push the pace – and the distance – so that you will feel you are working out hard. See page 70 for ideas on a training programme that includes walking.

Jogging

Introducing jogging for the first time in your routine can be a challenge, so start slowly and build the pace gradually. See page 72 for some tips on getting your jogging up and going!

Stepping

Using a step board (which you can get from good sports shops) is a great way to get cardio exercise. You can use the step indoors and build fun routines that will push your fitness level and challenge your co-ordination and concentration at the same time. With this kind of routine you can also put on some music to keep you motivated. If you want to do some outdoor stepping you can make use of steps in parks and other areas near you.

Circuits

One of the ideal ways to form a total-body workout is to include circuit training. See chapter 8 for some ideas on how you can include this in your weekly routine.

Check it's cardio

A very quick way to check if what you're doing is primarily cardio is to begin the training and then run through this checklist in your mind:

▶ Am I challenging the large muscle for the body part I am exercising – for example when exercising the legs, am I using the buttocks, hamstrings and/or quadriceps?

▶ Am I performing fairly repetitive movements that are rhythmical and sustained?

▶ Am I needing to breathe quite hard? Hard enough that I have to make sure I take a breath every other step, yet not so hard that I can't hold a conversation with someone or whistle to myself?

If your answer to the above three questions is yes, then you can be sure you are performing cardiovascular exercise.

Sports such as tennis, squash and baseball have elements of cardio work in them but, because of their stop–start nature, are not classic cardio workouts. Games such as rugby and football include cardio work and also include elements of anaerobic work – the intense kind of exercise performed above the level of a comfortable cardio pace, where you can feel you are pushing your body all out for results. A classic example of anaerobic exercise, used in many sports and pursuits, is sprinting.

Anaerobic exercise is a great way to add variation to a cardio workout and increase your fitness levels at the same time. Most cardio programmes include elements of anaerobic exercise to push the heart and lungs and muscles. It's important to remember, however, that anaerobic exercise is a high-risk activity. Because you are working the body at its outer limits, you must be careful to make sure you carry it out safely. Include this as part of your training, but only from time to time. Include it during weeks when you are feeling strong and when you have had the time to warm up and build up to that portion of the routine. Never begin a workout with anaerobic exercise.

Key cardio training points

There may be times when it is difficult to tell at what level of cardio you are performing and whether you are working hard enough or too hard. If you work too gently you may find you are not getting the results for the time you are putting in and if you work too hard you may exhaust yourself and become prone to injury. Use this calculation to figure out what your heart rate should be when training in order to get the most benefit.

The target heart rate calculation:

220 – your age = your maximum heart rate (figure A)

Example: 220 – 40 = 180

You don't want to work near your maximum heart rate as this forces your body into anaerobic rather than cardiovascular exercise. So, take two percentages of figure A: one at 55 per cent, the easier end of the scale (figure B); and one at 80 per cent, the tougher end of the training scale (figure C).

Example: 180 x 55 per cent = 99 (figure B)
180 x 80 per cent = 144 (figure C)

If you want to work at the lower end of the aerobic scale, your heart rate should match figure B or thereabouts. When you are upping the intensity of your session and aiming to push yourself, work at around figure C. Now you have the information you need, see page 62 for the correct way to measure your pulse during exercise to ensure you are working at the target level.

Your toning options

Toning is a very general term; what is really meant by the word 'toning' is the increase in endurance and strength of muscle tissue. To increase the strength of your muscles (and get the toned effect of strong, lean limbs) you have to put your muscles under stress. This means working them against resistance. If you try to push a wall down you are working your muscles by pushing them against something much stronger. Working your muscles, by moving through a range of movements, against resistance, is an even better way to tone them. Therefore in order to tone effectively you need to repeat muscle contractions against some form of resistance, whether it be pushing or pulling, working simply against gravity or using additional tools.

When you a lift a bag of shopping you are working your bicep muscles (at the front of the upper arm) against the resistance of the heavy bag. Every movement of bones in the body requires contraction of one set of muscles and stretching of an opposing set of muscles. Keep this process in mind as you think through the best way to tone areas of your body on which you wish to concentrate.

Use this book to put together an enjoyable routine that will tone the major muscles in your body in a variety of ways. As with cardio exercise, there is more than one way to achieve muscular tone, so pick and choose the workouts that appeal to you. These are the toning options included in this book.

Weight training

Weight training is one of the most conventional ways to build muscle. Using machines in a gym or lifting free weights allows you to make repeated contractions with different muscles in order to tire each individual muscle. Tiring the muscle is the key to seeing improvement; as your muscle is challenged, the body responds by building more fibrous, stronger – and thus more shapely – muscle tissue.

See chapter 7 for weight-training exercises you should consider incorporating in your workouts.

Kick-boxing

Kick-boxing involves lifting and extending the legs in a percussive and repeated fashion. While the focus of the routine is on kicking and punching an imaginary opponent, the muscles are being asked to contract repeatedly against the pull of gravity. Kick-boxing is a great example of a fun way to use your own body weight to increase your strength and muscle tone.

See chapter 7 for kick-boxing exercises you should consider incorporating in your workouts.

Circuit training

Circuit training can be used for muscle building as well as cardiovascular work. The benefit of this form of training is that you complete a variety of exercises within an allocated time, activating all the major muscle groups and keeping your mind busy while you concentrate on co-ordination, technique and preparing for the next station.

See chapter 8 for ideas for different circuit-training stations you can put into your programme so that your muscles are challenged and respond by becoming stronger and more defined.

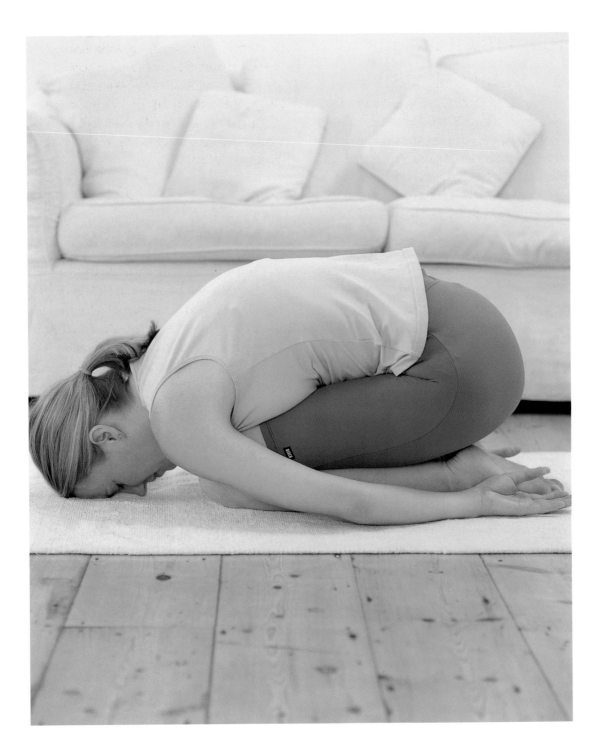

Your stretch and relaxation options

Stretching out isn't just about stretching your muscles but relaxing your whole body and mind. Stretching the muscles and focusing the mind are best done at both the beginning and end of a workout session. Many of the warm-up moves included in this book can be peformed as the cool-down phase.

At the end of a workout it's important to return the muscles to their pre-exercise state, so that they are no longer contracted but stretched back to their original length. In the same way you need to return your whole body to normality (after the intense concentration of exercise) and your mind to a calm state.

It is a good habit to get into winding down, calming and relaxing your body and mind after the physical busy-ness of an exercise routine. If you can work on slowing your thought process for a while so that for a few minutes you can feel some peace and calm, then you will feel really rejuven-ated. Training your mind not to rerun its constant inner dialogue can leave you feeling truly refreshed, like you've just had a mini holiday! But mind training, like muscle training, takes practice and application.

These are the stretching and relaxing options included in this book that will help train both body and mind.

Yoga

There are many different types of yoga, but all forms use a series of set movements as a way of stretching, toning and strengthening the body. Included in these pages are numerous yoga postures that can be used in all elements of your workout to enhance strength and posture and also to keep you sleek and flexible. Use the workout templates on pages 31–35 to drop in the elements you wish to include.

Pilates

Joseph Pilates put together a programme of movements in the first half of last century that revolutionised the way many people approached exercise and strength training. Used initially by physiotherapists and then dancers, Pilates has since won mainstream acceptance for its success in building core strength.

The body 'core' refers to the muscles of the back, sides and abdomen. The focus of Pilates moves is on working these muscles so that the body twists, turns and bends effortlessly. A strong body core means a back protected from stress, a flat stomach and ease of movement.

Follow the Pilates basics in this book (such as pages 96–97) to reap the benefits!

Chi Gung

This non-contact martial art is closely related to Tai Chi and uses slow, controlled movements to harness and enhance energy – the 'Chi'. Chi Gung movements calm and restore balance, helping you to wind down, or alternatively harness the energy you need to get going.

The Chi Gung moves in this book (see page 54) introduce you to the concept of tuning into your energy to get the most out of any workout.

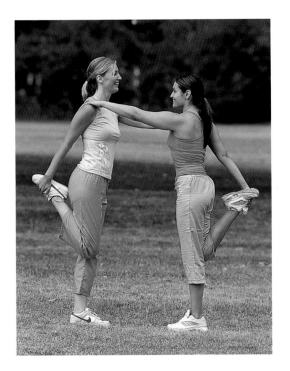

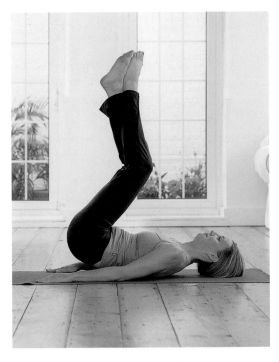

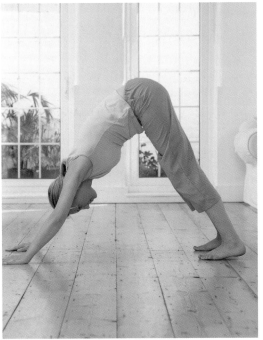

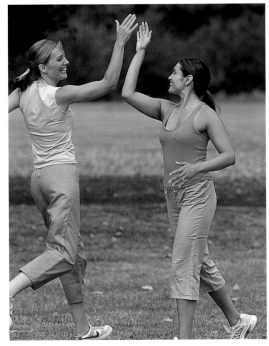

Your workout templates

You may like to photocopy these templates and use them for structuring your own workouts. Use them as a tool or prompt for outlining which elements you will incorporate in a workout in order to achieve the benefits outlined in chapter 1. This is where it all comes together.

Enter here the areas of fitness you are most lacking in (from page 13): ....

....

....

Enter here your main focus in your training (from the quiz on page 22): ....

....

....

Enter the time needed to achieve the above criteria: ....

....

....

Break down the above time into the blocks that will fit into your schedule (see the chart on page 23): ....

....

....

....

Re-read page 14 'What elements should a home fitness programme include?' to check there isn't some other element of the fitness equation you haven't considered and might need to include. Now you can plot the actual workout into the chart over the page.

This month's main goal: ....

WEEK 1

DAY AND TIME	LENGTH OF SESSION	TYPE OF EXERCISE

WEEK 2

DAY AND TIME	LENGTH OF SESSION	TYPE OF EXERCISE

WEEK 3

DAY AND TIME	LENGTH OF SESSION	TYPE OF EXERCISE

WEEK 4

DAY AND TIME	LENGTH OF SESSION	TYPE OF EXERCISE

Sample workouts

Here are some sample weekly workout charts developed for specific goals. Be inspired by them and make them your own. Note that each workout session, other than one specifically aimed at relaxation, begins with a 5-minute warm-up and ends with a 5-minute cool-down.

Goal: Weight loss

DAY AND TIME	LENGTH OF SESSION	TYPE OF EXERCISE
Monday, 7.30 a.m.	**30 minutes**	**Kick-boxing**
Wednesday, 6.30 p.m.	**30 minutes**	**Low-impact workout**
Saturday, 10 a.m.	**60 minutes**	**Walking and mind relaxation**

Goal: Toning the stomach

DAY AND TIME	LENGTH OF SESSION	TYPE OF EXERCISE
Tuesday, 12 noon	**30 minutes**	**Express abs workout**
Wednesday, 5 p.m.	**30 minutes**	**Core conditioning**
Friday, 12 noon	**15 minutes**	**Yoga abs**

Goal: Shaping arms and legs

DAY AND TIME	LENGTH OF SESSION	TYPE OF EXERCISE
Sunday, 6 p.m.	30 minutes	Walking
Tuesday, 8 a.m.	15 minutes	Triceps routine
Thursday, 8 a.m.	15 minutes	Biceps routine

Goal: Stretch and relaxation

DAY AND TIME	LENGTH OF SESSION	TYPE OF EXERCISE
Monday, 7 a.m.	10 minutes	Yoga breathing
Wednesday, 5 p.m.	30 minutes	Stretching the spine
Thursday, 7 a.m.	10 minutes	Mind relaxation

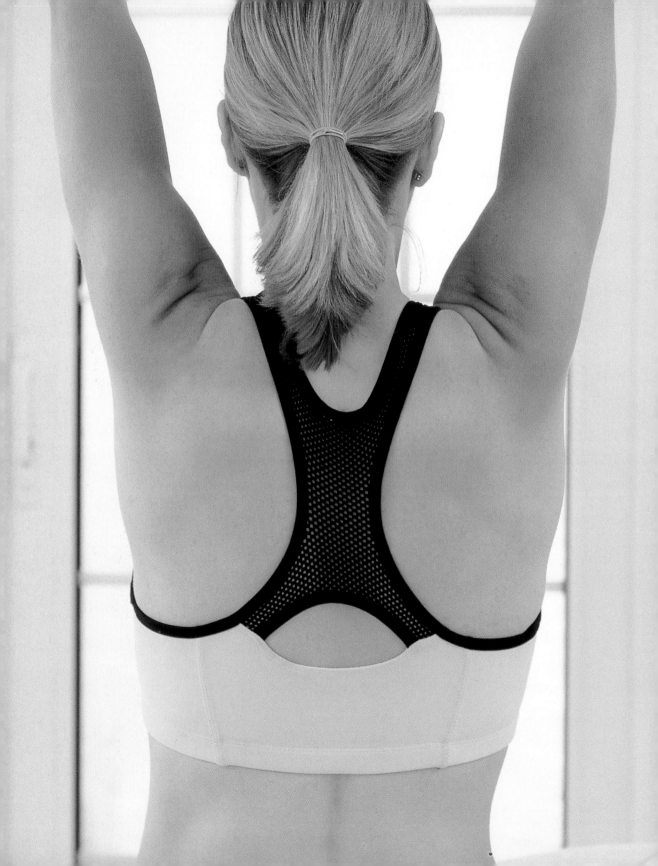

chapter 3
the warm-up

It's time to get down to the nuts and bolts of building your own workout. While a machine-based workout can get boring, doing the same thing day in day out, your home workout programme is bound only by your imagination. Think of your workouts as a pick-and-mix bag of goodies. Practise each move until you feel confident, then choose which moves you want to incorporate in the day's workout. Whatever kind of programme you have put together for yourself, and whatever goals you have in mind, it is important that you always start your workout with a warm-up.

Readying your mind and body

Warming up is simply a way of readying your mind and body for exercise. If you have rushed in from work at the end of the day or have been out gardening and decided to come inside to start your home workout, your body and mind will need preparation. Moving straight into complicated exercises could lead to injuries and reduce the effectiveness of your programme. As you warm up, you build your body temperature so that your muscles are ready for action, your brain is engaged and you can begin to concentrate completely on what you are doing. A good warm-up will help you put your worries aside and help you focus on your time for exercise.

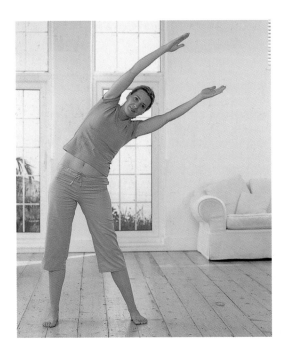

The advantages of a good warm-up:

▶ As your core body temperature increases, the blood vessels dilate, which allows good flow of blood to all areas and reduces the work for the heart.

▶ As the temperature of the muscles increases, they become more pliant and are able to contract forcefully and relax readily. This guards against muscle strain. It also means the muscles will be at their optimum for working intensely and gaining strength and stamina.

▶ Increased blood temperature is thought to allow a greater release of oxygen into the working muscles so you have a greater potential for available energy.

▶ As you warm up the body, hormonal changes occur which allow more carbohydrates and fatty acids to be available for energy production.

▶ As your body prepares for activity, so does your mind. Practise concentration and leave all the problems of the day behind you as you focus purely on the task at hand. Not only will this mean your workout is concentrated and thoughtful but you will also end your session feeling mentally refreshed after having thought of nothing else for the duration.

A warm-up routine can take many forms and there are no set movements that must be included. The key is using all the major body parts to limber up, warm up in temperature and prepare for action. Have a read through the pages that follow for ideas to include in the warm-up phase of your workout.

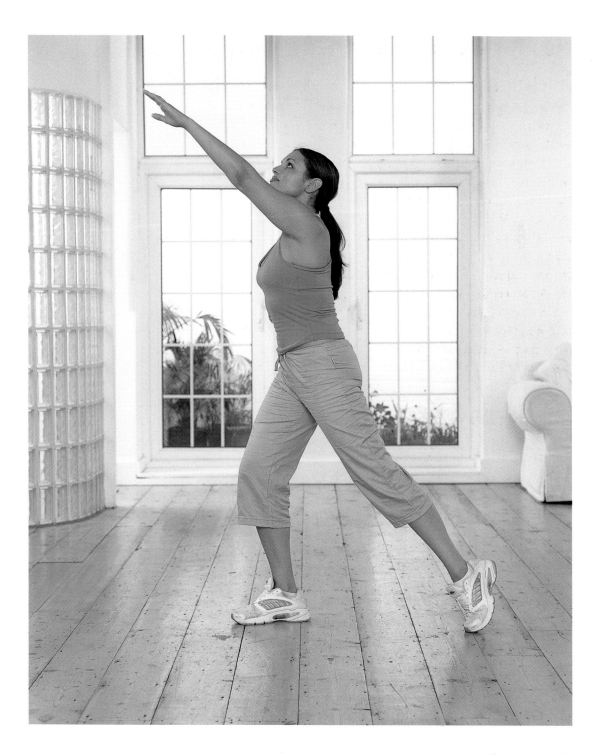

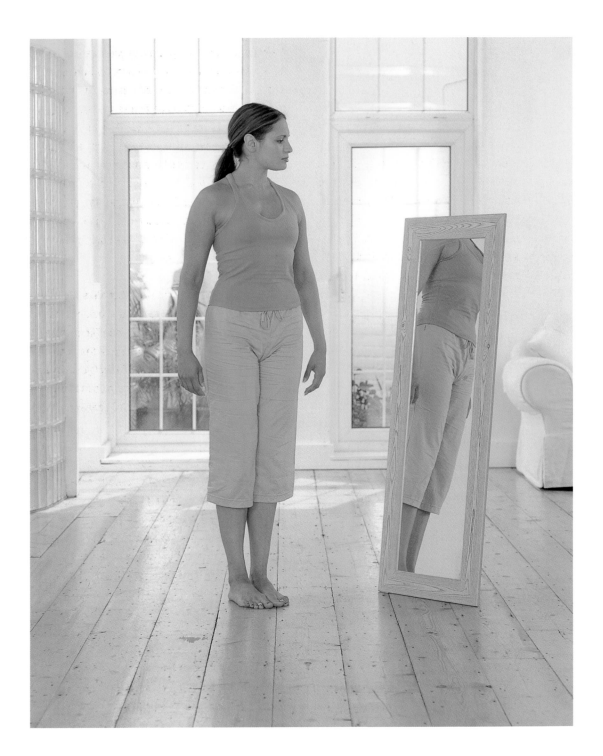

Establishing good posture

One of the quickest ways to improve your appearance and muscle tone is to work first on your posture. Posture is the body's alignment or stacking system of head resting on shoulders, ribcage sitting on hips and transferring the weight through to the feet. Sometimes, due to injuries, muscular imbalances or simply stress, the body's alignment can be altered and start to cause problems. If at the beginning of each of your workouts you spend some time re-establishing good posture, you will start to see and feel a difference in the way you hold yourself.

THE YOGA MOUNTAIN POSE

This yoga basic is a great way to check your posture and establish good alignment before you begin further movements. In yoga this position starts and finishes all the standing postures of the yoga workout, bringing the body back to perfect alignment each time.

✳ Stand in front of a mirror so that you can watch what is happening with your body.

✳ Stand with your feet together. Big toes, ankles and heels should be touching.

✳ Take a moment here to become aware of where you are balancing on your feet. Are you inclined to roll in a little on your feet (this is called 'pronation')? Are you inclined to roll outwards on your feet (this is called 'supination')? These two

tendencies alone can you make you aware of some basic imbalance that you may need to work on. Continue to stand very still and make sure that your weight is evenly distributed across the ball, outer toes and heel of each foot. If you feel some imbalance, don't worry, just shift your weight slightly to reaffirm the correct positions and as you continue to use this pose your body will start to learn the correct balance. Working on your posture like this might seem simple but sometimes it is difficult to beat those bad habits. This will also help prevent knee and ankle problems.

✳ Next, concentrate on your shoulders. Roll them backwards and squeeze the shoulder blades together slightly. This should not look like a military soldier's stance; it is an opening up of the chest and upper breastbone: you should feel your ribcage lift. Many people have a tendency to round their upper back, dropping the chin and concaving the chest. Try to avoid this.

✳ Now concentrate on your lower back. Turn face-on to the mirror. Check you are not overarching your lower back, leaning back on your heels with your tummy thrust forward. If you do spot this tendency, pull your coccyx (tailbone) down towards the floor and tilt your hip bones very slightly up towards you. Don't overdo it by contracting the abdominals, though. The feeling should be of your tailbone pressing down to the floor and the top of your head lifting up to the ceiling.

✳ Take a couple of seconds in this perfect position to let your body register how it feels. Remember these feelings so that you can come back to this for the start of each workout.

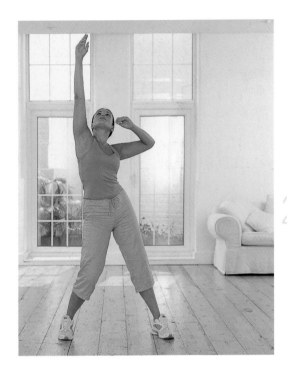

Step and reach 8–10 times on each side. Keep the move flowing and gentle like a dance movement.

You will feel the sides of your body stretching – right the way from the hip up into the ribcage and the side of the lattisimus dorsi (see page 16) to the shoulders.

HIP ROTATIONS AND REVOLUTIONS

Stand with your feet hip-width apart and hands on your hips. Bend your knees and press your hands to the left to send your hips to the left. Now use the pressure of your hands to push your hips to the right. Press from side to side to feel a loosening of your hips.

From the hip rotations, straighten your legs and again press your hips from side to side. Press your hips forwards and backwards and then into a circular movement.

Move your hips all the way around in a large circle, first one way and then the other. Repeat 8–10 times. You will feel the joints of your hips and sides of the waist being mobilised and starting to free up.

Mobilisation

Once you have established good postural habits, start to move around a little. Some gentle mobilisation exercises are a great way to get your body prepared for further exercise. Try these simple moves to get your body in the mood!

STRETCH AND REACH

Stand with your feet hip-width apart. Reach both hands into the air. Now step on to one foot and reach with the same arm even higher. As you step on to this foot, bend the knee so that you are leaning slightly to one side. Now step on to the other foot and reach with the other arm, leaning into the bend.

TRAINING TIP
To really mobilise the hip joints and the waist, swing your hips out to all directions as wide as you can. Also vary the speed, performing faster and slower rotations.

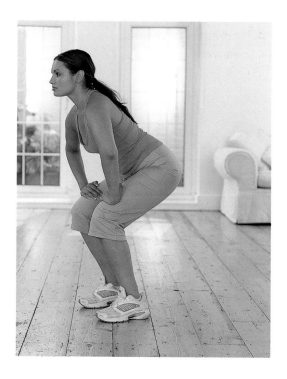

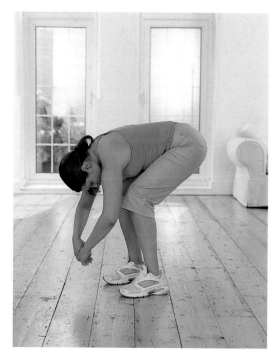

3 SQUAT BENDS

✳ Stand with your feet hip-width apart and bend both knees, pushing your backside out well behind you.

✳ Lower your torso downwards, keeping your legs where they are. Place your hands on your knees, allowing your upper body to fold over your legs. Hold for 10 seconds.

✳ Relax your neck muscles, letting your head hang, and allow your arms to rest on the floor. You will feel your lower back release.

✳ Slowly roll up through your spine, uncurling your back until your upper body is straight and you can push through your legs to finish straight and tall.

TRAINING TIPS

When you perform a true squat bend, you bend until your thighs are parallel with the floor. You might not be able to get this low when you start out, but if you lean your back against a wall for extra support, you should get the best stretch.

Keep your weight over your heels as you lower yourself down. This really targets the buttock muscles.

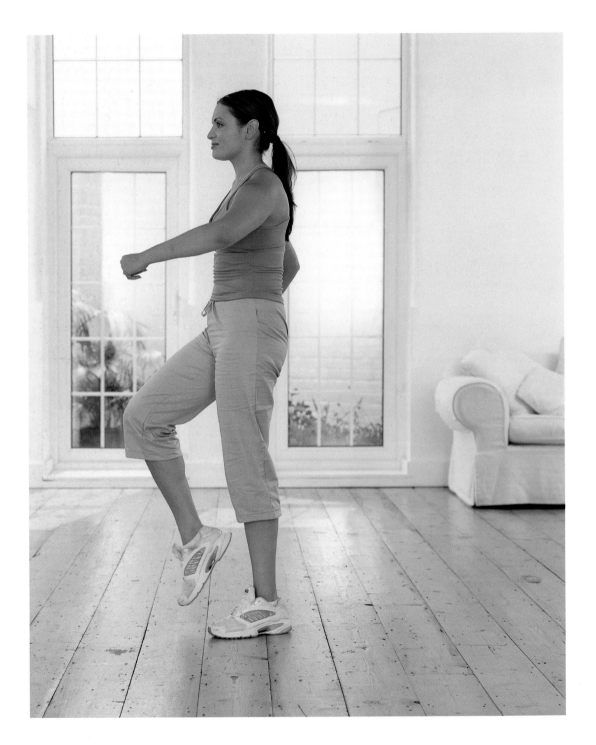

Thorough warm-up

This routine comprises more general movement – it is a way to get moving, increase your body temperature and start to get into the idea of working hard. Try putting on some music for these moves – as loud as the neighbours can bear – and start grooving!

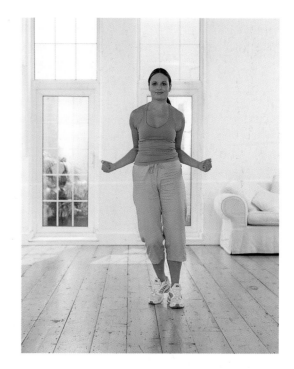

1 MARCHING OUT

✳ Begin by marching on the spot, in time to the music and pumping your arms at the same time. Keep lifting your knees and pumping your arms higher and higher.

✳ Make sure you roll your feet along the floor from the toes through to heels. This ensures your feet get warmed up too.

✳ You will feel your breathing become heavier as you march faster and lift your knees higher.

2 SIDE TO SIDE

✳ Move from marching on the spot to a side-to-side step movement. Step to the left and touch your feet together, then step back to the right and bring your feet together again. Use the music to get into this move; as you touch your feet together, sink into it, bending your knees a little more each time. Swing your arms in time.

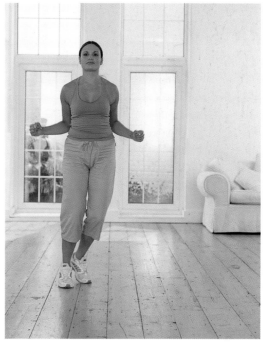

✳ You will notice as you go from one move to another that your breathing becomes slightly heavier because your body is having to work that much harder. You should also notice your body getting warmer and warmer.

3 LUNGE

✳ Go back to the marching again for several minutes and take some deep breaths. Breathe in through the nose and out through the mouth slowly and purposefully.

✳ Now from the march, as you pick up one knee, press your leg further behind you so that your back leg is straight and your front leg is bent. Swing both arms out in front of you to help keep your balance, as one foot reaches out the back.

✳ You will feel the front of your hip stretching a little as you reach the leg behind. You will also be warming up the leg that is doing the bending. Repeat 12 times, changing legs each time.

4 TRY A SEQUENCE

Once you have the feel of the above marching, side-to-side and lunge moves, try combining them to form a mini sequence that fits to the music you are listening to.

A suggestion might be: marching on the spot for 2 minutes, stepping side to side for 2 minutes, back into the marching for 1 minute, then on to 3 minutes of backward lunging. Bring it back to the marching for a further minute and finish with a minute of stepping side to side. In this way you can 'dance' for 10 minutes, enjoying the music and warming up your body in a fun, relaxed way.

TRAINING TIPS

Be careful that the bent knee stays directly above the foot. Your weight should be pushing back on the straight leg behind.

Even at this early stage in your workout, reminding yourself to breathe deeply is important. Your body needs more and more oxygen as you exercise, so train yourself to breathe regularly and deeply from the beginning.

Perform these moves with energy and conviction. As you limber up and start to enjoy yourself you can make the moves larger. Try to lift your legs higher and punch your arms harder. This will get your body ready for the higher-impact exercise to come.

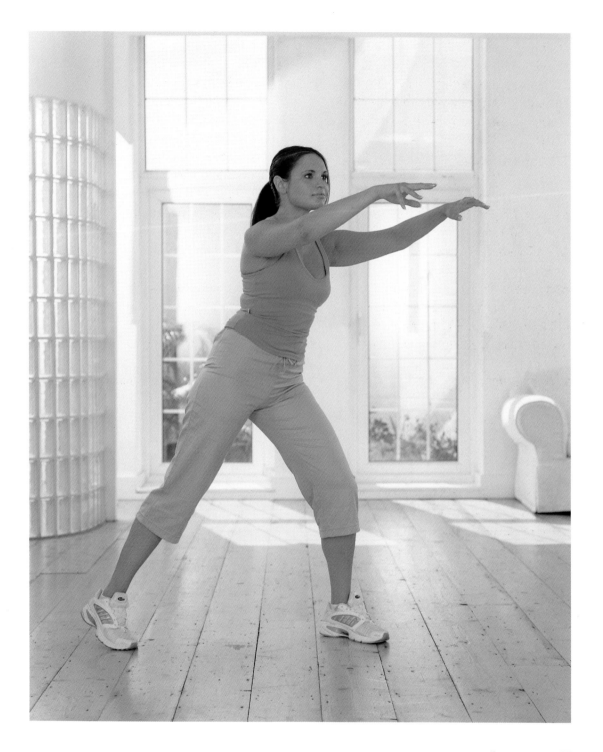

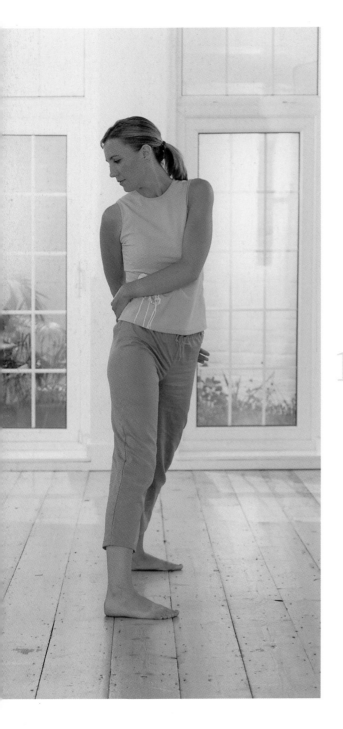

Tibetan rites warm-up exercises

Practised and expounded by Tibetan monks as excellent exercises for rejuvenating health and promoting longevity, the Tibetan rites exercises comprise a programme of unusual bending and twisting moves. The core programme of exercises is not suitable for the uninitiated and requires instruction from a trainer; however, there are five Tibetan rites warm-up moves that are simple to perform and a great way to loosen up your muscles and warm up your limbs. Try these unusual moves and if you like them, incorporate them into your weekly workout regime.

1 SWINGING MOVE

✳ Stand with your feet hip-width apart, knees slightly bent.

✳ Keep the bottom half of your body stationary and swing your arms around your body, letting the swing of your arms pull the top part of your body around with them. Relax your arms totally, allowing them to slap against your back and shoulders as they swing. You should feel your waist twisting and loosening.

✳ Next, extend the swing and let it pull your hips and the tops of your legs into it as well. Be careful not to twist at the knees, however. Keep your toes on the floor, but allow your heels to lift off as you twist.

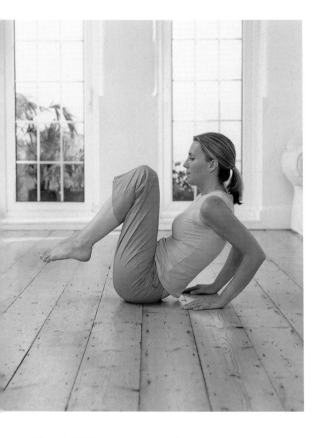

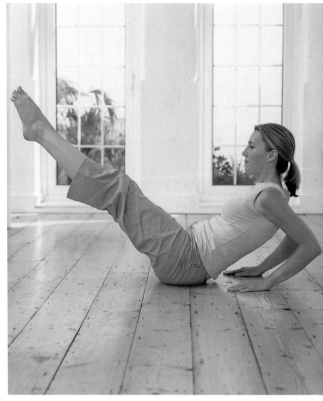

2 LEG EXTENSION

✳ Sit on your bottom with hands behind you.

✳ Lean back and pull both knees into your chest. Keep your knees together.

✳ Slowly extend your legs, keeping your knees together all the while, until they are almost straight. Hold for 5 seconds, then bend your legs back in.

✳ Repeat three or four times, making sure you feel the work in your stomach muscles.

TRAINING TIPS

If you start to feel your back muscles tightening while performing this exercise, rest then try again, concentrating on contracting your abdominals.

The higher you lift your legs towards your head, the easier the exercise is on the abdominals. As you lower your legs you will feel greater stress on your abdominals. Lower your legs for a more challenging stretch as you start to feel stronger.

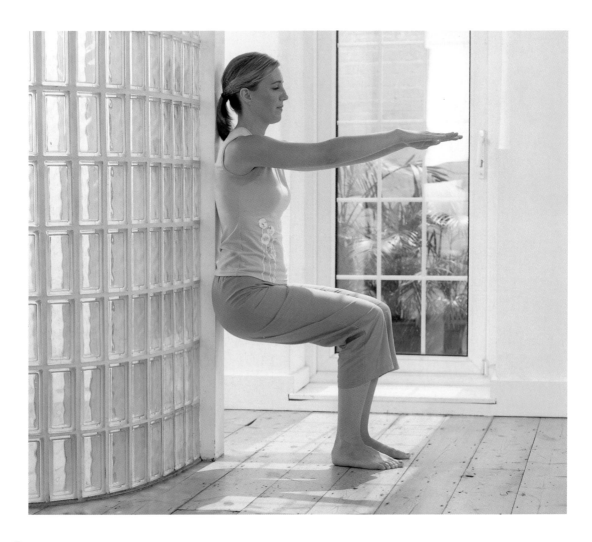

3 SQUAT PRACTICE AGAINST A WALL

✳ Stand with your back against a wall and with your feet hip-width apart.

✳ Bend your knees, pressing your buttocks to the wall, extending your arms out in front of you or resting your hands on your thighs.

✳ Slide down the wall slowly, keeping your back straight and holding your stomach in, until your thighs are parallel with the floor. Hold for a few seconds.

✳ Slowly press down through your legs and straighten up. Repeat four or five times.

Yoga warm-up

Another way to think of a warm-up is to think of readying the body for exercise by releasing tension. When your body is full of tension and stiffness from a busy day, you may not feel like exercising, but performing some simple moves to help you relax will get you in the mood for exercise.

Of the many benefits of yoga, one of the most important is its ability to help you relax and refocus. Yoga involves a series of carefully balanced postures that are performed rhythmically and with the intentional use of the breath. Learning basic yoga breathing technique is a great way to warm up and focus your mind.

THE COMPLETE YOGA BREATH

✷ Sit with your legs crossed on the floor. If you have done yoga before and would like to sit in full or half lotus, do so; however, just sitting cross-legged is perfect for now. Keep your spine upright and eyes focused straight ahead.

✷ Allow your shoulders to relax.

✷ Lengthen the back of your neck so that your chin drops slightly.

✷ Place both hands on your stomach.

✷ Breathe in through the nose and out slowly, also through the nose. As you begin to breathe in, the first thing that should happen is that your abdomen should expand. In other words, focus the breath right down into the stomach.

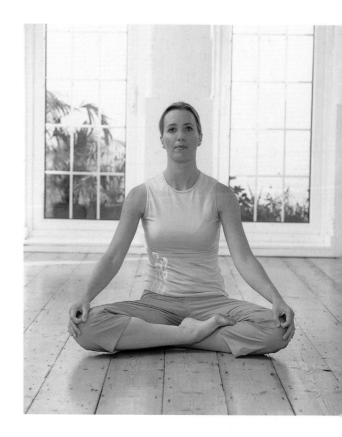

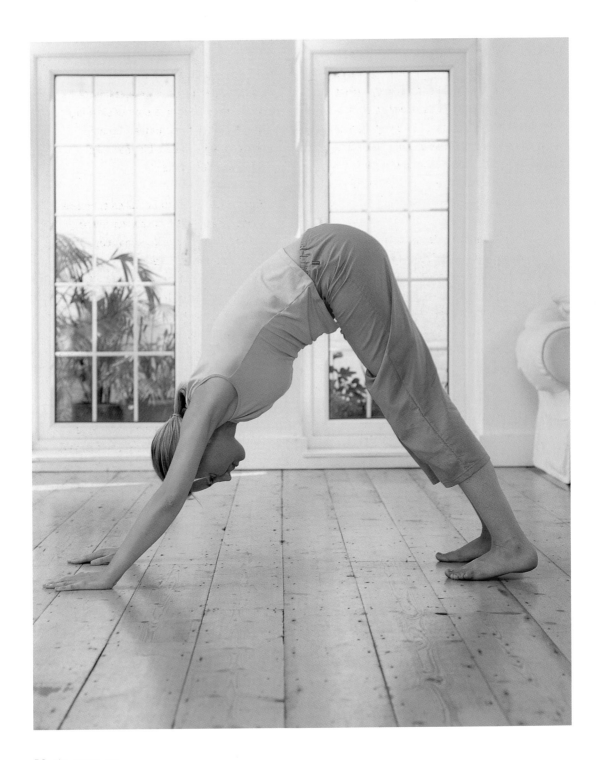

❋ Once you have mastered focusing the breath in the stomach, turn your attention to your ribcage. Move your breath to expand your ribcage. Place your hands around your ribcage, with your fingers splayed out and fingertips just touching. As your breath reaches and expands your ribcage area, you should be able to see your hands being pulled apart. Concentrate on this breathing for a minute or so.

❋ Turn your attention to focusing the breath on filling your chest cavity. Feel the whole area expand. Concentrate on this breathing for a minute.

❋ On the outward breath (still through the nose), concentrate on contracting first the stomach area, then the ribcage and finally the chest to expel the last of each breath.

2 **DOWNWARD DOG**

❋ Start off on your hands and knees on the floor.

❋ Curl your toes under and straighten your legs slowly, pushing your buttocks up into the air and inhaling as you do so.

❋ Press backwards on your hands, so that you are pressing your chest toward the floor.

❋ Hold for a few breaths and then lower gently back to your knees. Repeat three or four times.

Chi Gung warm-up

Chi Gung is a system of movements which are generally considered to be the foundation of Chinese martial arts. The exercises evolved from the first set of movements taught by the Indian missionary Bodhidharma on his arrival at the monasteries of China. The focus is on release of the 'Chi' – the energy – from all over the body. It is a regime with many similarities to yoga, especially with its emphasis on the breath. Following is an explanation of the Chi Gung approach to breathing, which you can consider incorporating into your daily workouts. There is also an example of a popular and very effective Chi Gung exercise: hugging a tree.

Three styles of Chi breathing

Chi breathing incorporates different styles of inhaling and expelling the breath. Three of these breathing styles are 'natural breathing', 'Taoist reverse breathing' and 'Buddhist breathing'.

Natural breathing is the breathing you do when concentrating on a particular physical move – the natural way you inhale and exhale when focusing on something else. This method is used when a student of Chi Gung first begins to learn the Chi moves and needs to concentrate on the physical movement sequence before adding a breathing element.

Taoist reverse breathing uses the method of pulling in on the stomach when you inhale and relaxing the muscles as you exhale. This method is used for moving the Chi forcefully through the body to achieve specific results – for example, for the purposes of muscle strengthening or for healing in a particular part of the body.

The most common method employed during Chi Gung exercises, however, is Buddhist breathing. This breathing method is identical to yoga breathing, where the breath is concentrated first in the stomach, then ribcage, followed by the chest cavity (see pages 51 and 53).

HUG A TREE

✳ This Chi Gung exercise is exactly as the name suggests: a pose where you stand as though hugging a tree! Stand with your feet hip-width apart and with your knees slightly bent.

✳ Take your arms out in front of you with hands apart but palms facing each other.

✳ Use Buddhist, or yoga, breathing and start to count how many seconds each breath takes.

✳ Your aim is to make each breath last longer. Try to breathe in for a count of four then breathe out for a count of four. Concentrate on making each breath longer than the one before and keeping the inhalations and exhalations even in length. With practice you will be able to elongate the breath to a count of 10 or 15 or more.

> ### TRAINING TIP
> As you develop your skills with this exercise, bend your knees further until your thighs are parallel with the floor. This increases the work on your thighs as well as the demand for oxygen.

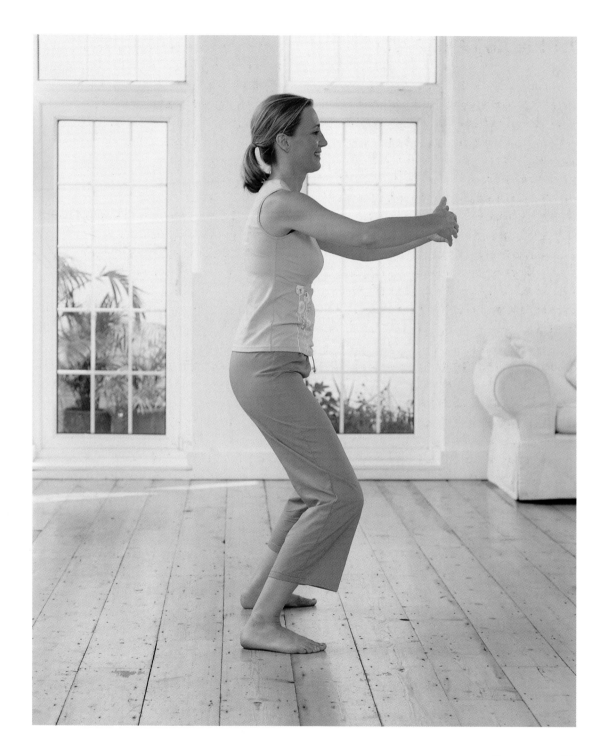

Express stretch

It is now widely considered unnecessary to perform lengthy stretches after a warm-up and before a main workout. It is better to keep the body warm and to perform what's called the developmental stretching at the end of the session. It is, however, beneficial to do some short stretches of the main muscle groups that ready the body for further action without letting the body cool down too much.

Perform each of these stretches by holding the position for 8–10 seconds and then moving on to the next one.

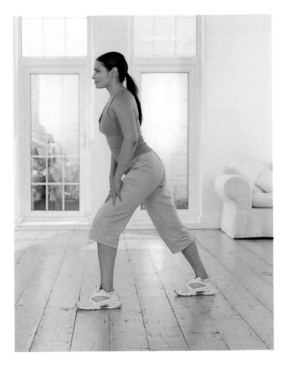

1 CALF EXPRESS

✱ Stand with one leg straight and directly behind you, foot facing forward, and with the other leg bent.

✱ Press back the heel into the floor and lean forward to feel a stretch at the back of the calf of the straight leg. Hold, then swap legs and repeat.

2 ACHILLES EXPRESS

✱ Stand on the edge of a step.

✱ Lean forward slightly and allow one heel to sink below the line of the step. Hold. This stretches out both the calf muscles and the Achilles tendon.

✱ Slowly lift the heel to come out of the stretch and repeat with the other foot.

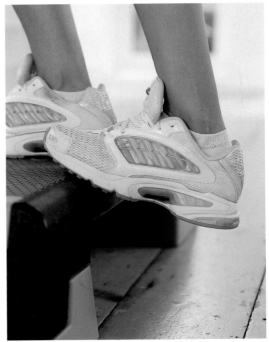

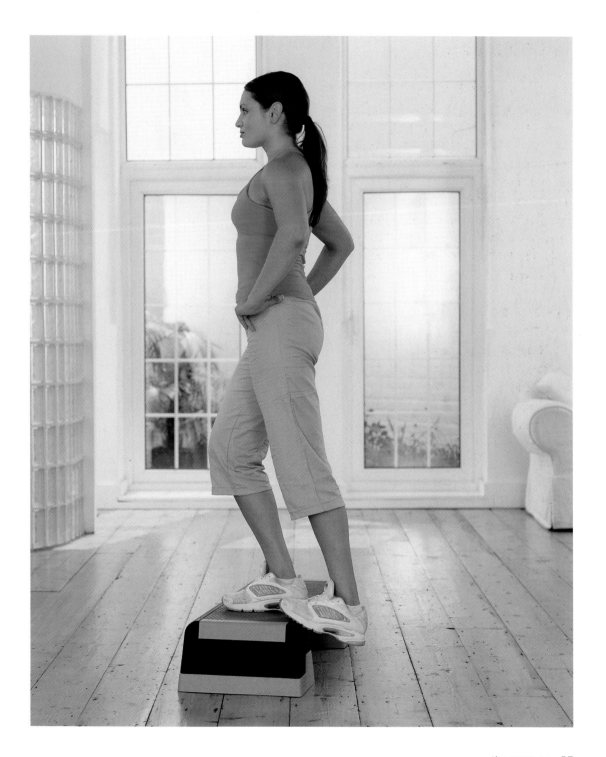

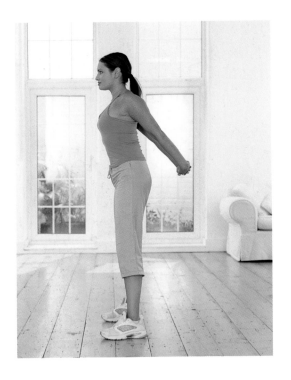

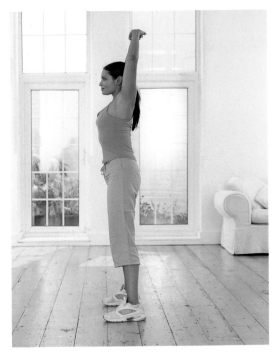

3 CHEST EXPRESS

✳ Stand with your feet hip-width apart and clasp your hands behind your back.

✳ Now straighten and lift your arms up a little way. You will feel an opening out and a stretching across the front of the chest, in your pectoral muscles. Hold.

4 SHOULDER EXPRESS

✳ Stand with your feet hip-width apart and this time link both hands above your head. Lift as high up as you can to feel a stretch up through the body.

✳ Now gently press your hands backwards. You should feel a stretch in the shoulder joints. Hold.

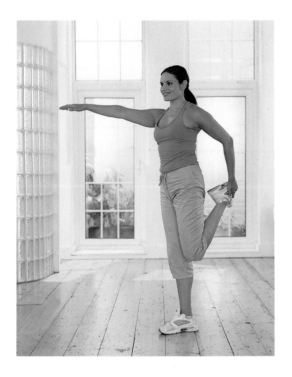

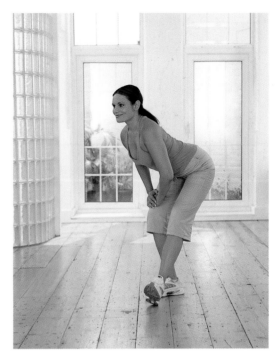

5 QUAD EXPRESS

✳ Stand near a wall or hold the back of a chair if you need the balance support for this stretch. Standing straight on one leg, bend the knee of the other leg, lifting the leg behind you. Grasp the foot of the bent leg with the matching hand.

✳ Press the heel of your foot in toward the buttock. Push your hips forward as far as they will go and hold your tummy in. Hold. You will feel a release or a stretch in the front of the thigh, along your quadriceps muscles. Repeat with the other leg.

6 HAM EXPRESS

✳ Start in a standing position. Push one leg out straight in front of you and bend the back leg. Your weight should be supported on the bent back leg.

✳ Push your buttocks behind you and bring your chest forward over the straight leg. Bend your upper body, supporting your weight with your hands on the thigh of your bent leg. Hold. You should feel a good stretch at the back of the thigh on the straight leg. You are working on the powerful hamstring group here.

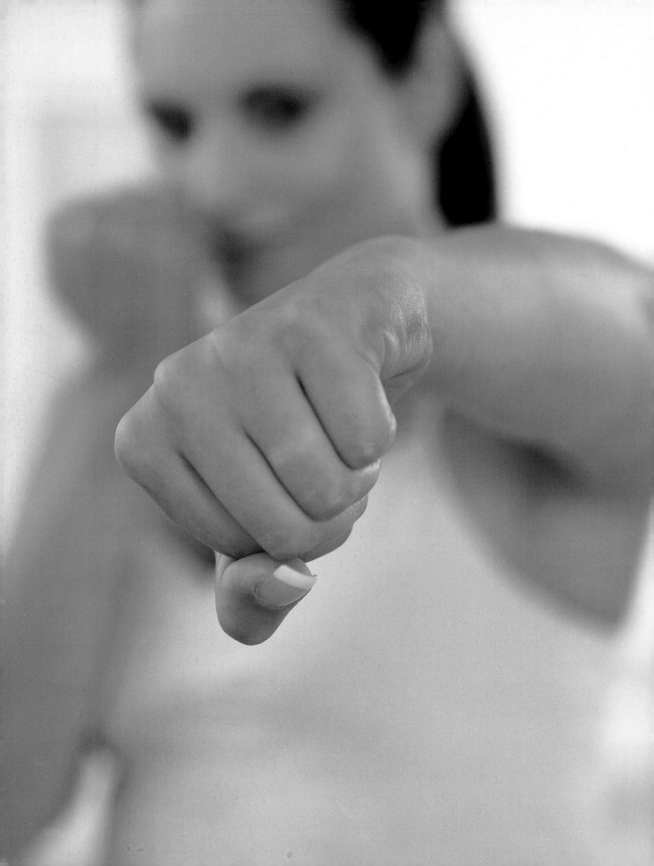

chapter 4

your cardiovascular workouts

There are two great things about aerobic movement. Firstly, it works out your heart and lungs, challenging them to give your body more oxygen and therefore making them stronger and more effective. This helps give you more energy in everyday life. Secondly, as you keep the rhythmical, large-muscle movements going, you start to burn fat for energy, leading to a slimmer, fitter you!

Pulse check

Back in chapter 1 we looked at a useful formula for indicating the training zone you need to be working within for different levels of activity. At this stage of your workout, as you begin the aerobic exercise section, it's important to be able to check your pulse and read the rate correctly. This means you can ensure you are working at the exact intensity you planned.

Checking your pulse at rest

Find the soft area on the inside of your wrist below the base of your thumb and next to the tendons that run up your forearm. Press two fingers (not a thumb) lightly on this area. You will feel the pulse of blood pushing through the veins. Count the number of pulses for one minute. Your resting pulse rate simply gives you an indication of what your heart is doing at times when you are not exercising.

Checking your pulse during the cardiovascular session

During the peak activity time of your cardio workout, check your pulse. At this stage, do not count the pulses for a whole minute, as this will give an inaccurate reading since your pulse rate will drop during this time. Instead, count the pulses over a period of just six seconds. Times your calculation by 10 (an easy calculation even when you're sweating!) to get your active pulse rate.

What to do with this information

By comparing your resting and active pulse rates you can see how hard you are working during your cardio session. If you are aiming for a light workout on a particular day, you will want to keep your pulse rate in the 55–65 per cent range for your age (see page 26). If you are really aiming to push your cardio work, then you are looking for your pulse to be in the 75–85 per cent range and to keep it there.

A true resting pulse

Your true resting pulse is actually the number of pulses you can count when you first wake up in the morning. If you have bounced out of bed, rushed around and had several cups of coffee, then taking your pulse count at this point won't indicate your true resting pulse. When you wake up, find your watch and your pulse, and time the count for one minute – all before you get out of bed. This indicates your true resting pulse.

You may like to keep a record of your pulse rates so that you can track your fitness levels over months and years. Take a reading once a month. As you get fitter and stronger you should notice your pulse getting slower (as your heart is getting more powerful).

What is a fit pulse?

A fit pulse is in the range of 50–60. An average to fair fitness level will display a pulse rate of 61–75. Poor fitness will display a pulse rate of 75+. Professional athletes have pulse rates as low as 35!

Low-impact workout

These are some nuts-and-bolt ideas for a low-impact workout routine. The term 'low-impact' refers to the fact that there is less jumping off the ground with two feet and more walking- and hopping-type moves. This produces less impact on the body – a good thing if you are recovering from an injury, for example. It also means that the routine will probably keep you in the lower range of your target training zone. When you add higher-impact moves, not only does it increase the stress on the body but it also pushes the heart rate up. Both types of workout intensity have their place in an all-round fitness programme and are great to add variety to your training.

Many people prefer low impact, with less bouncy moves, because it is less jarring on the body. However, low-impact work doesn't always mean low energy levels. You can still put lots of energy into the shape and emphasis of the moves as you engage in a low-impact workout.

For this routine you may need to learn the moves first and then, with music playing, begin to combine the moves in a way that pleases you.

Don't forget to vary the view as you move – face the wall then face the door, perform some moves coming forwards and others moving backwards. Make it a dance! There are no right and wrong moves to add to an aerobic workout, as long as it keeps you moving, keeps your muscles working and keeps you breathing.

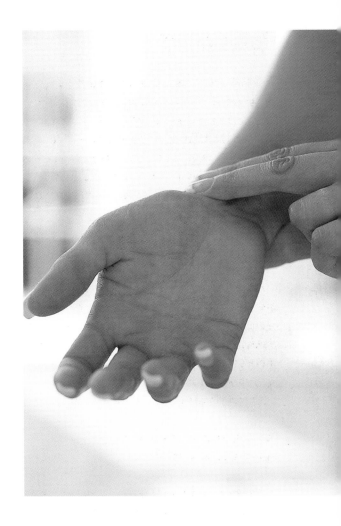

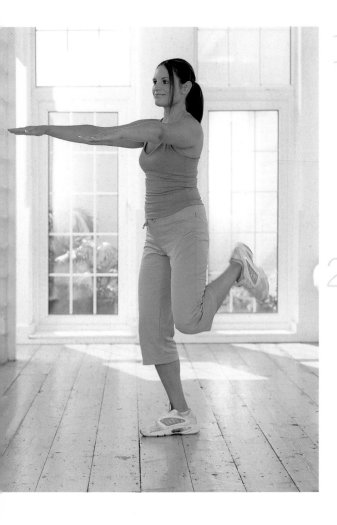

1 HOPSCOTCH

✳ Jump on to two feet and then hop on to one. Keep your eyes fixed straight ahead.

> ### TRAINING TIP
> Hop on to alternate feet and swing your arms in time to the movement.

2 LUNGE TWIST

✳ From the hopscotch move, reach your right leg out straight to the side, turning slightly to your left and keeping your weight on your bent left leg.

✳ Reach your right arm straight across your body in the direction you have turned.

✳ Alternate legs and build up a punching momentum that will help get your breathing going.

> ### TRAINING TIPS
> Punch with energy and twist with vigour.
>
> Feel the rhythm and make this move into a dance step!

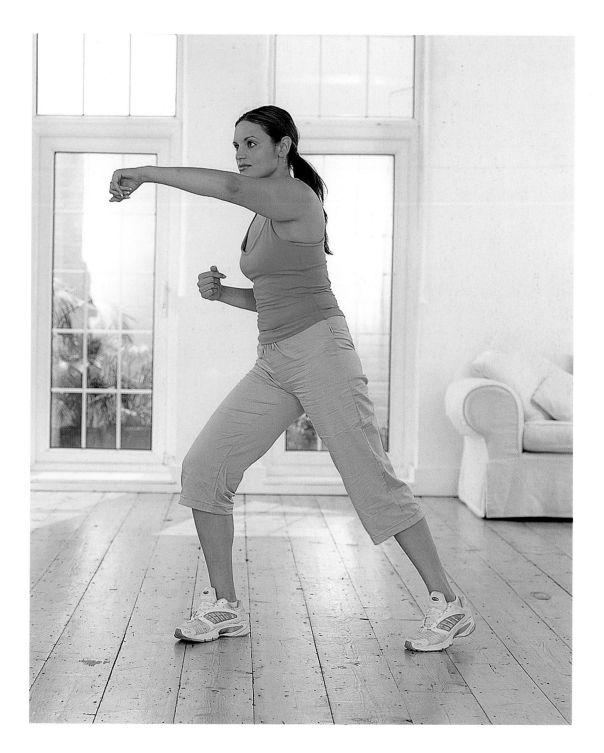

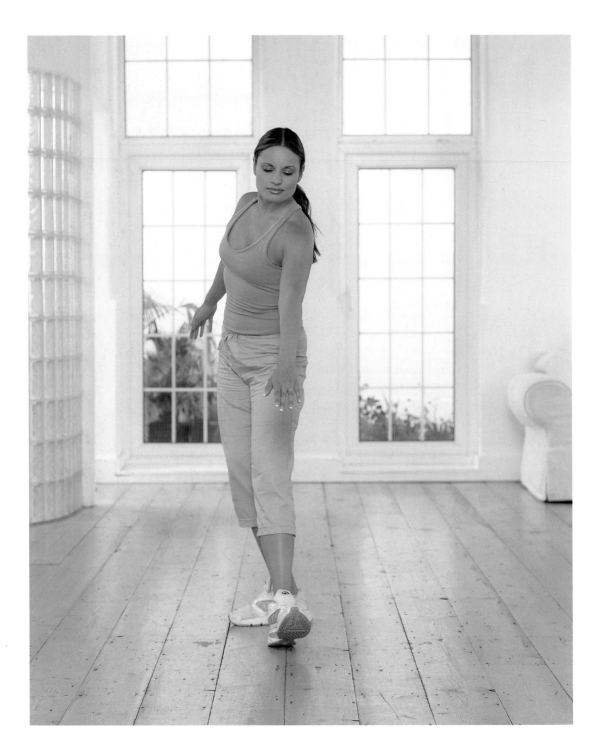

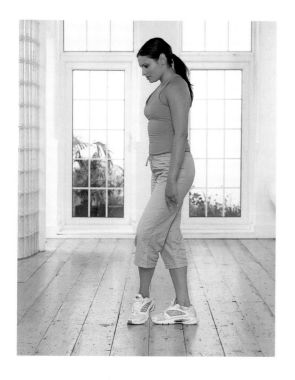

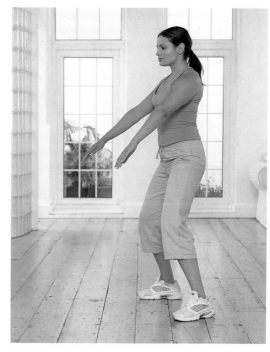

GRAPEVINE

This is a great upbeat move that forms part of any aerobics class at the gym.

✳ Start with your feet together. First, step to the side with your left foot.

✳ Step the right foot behind the left – both knees should be bent.

✳ Third, step to the side with your left foot again, so that you are moving across the room.

✳ Finally, jump and pull both feet together. Repeat, this time beginning with your right foot.

TRAINING TIP

Once you have got the hang of where your feet need to move for the grapevine, and can move easily from one side to the other, add some arm movements to get your top half working. You could also add weights to your arms and pump them in the air to work out different arm muscles.

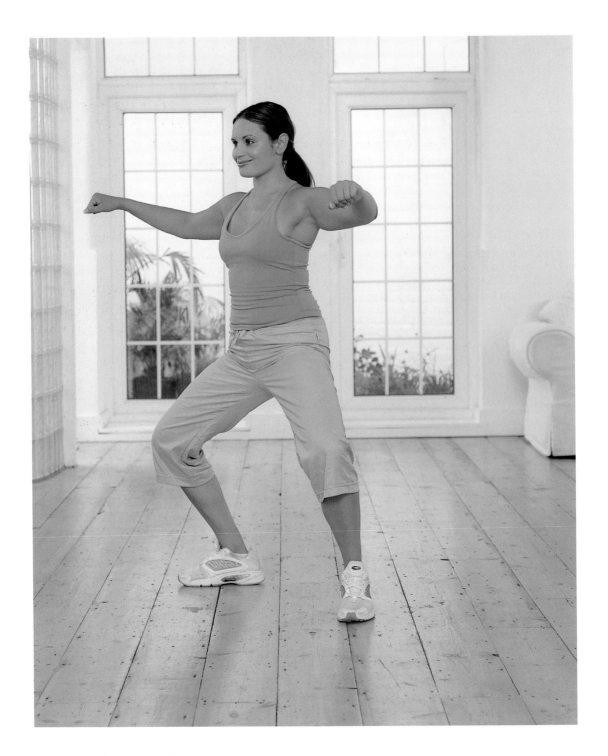

4 HALF JACKS

✻ This is a low-impact version of jumping jacks. Start with your feet together.

✻ Take one foot out to the side and, as it presses into the floor, bend both knees into a wide squat. Lift your arms out to the side, elbows slightly bent, as your legs bend.

✻ Push off with both feet and jump to the centre. Repeat, this time stepping to the opposite side.

> ### TRAINING TIP
> Perform 8–10 half jacks on each side after a couple of grapevine moves.

5 SPOT JOGGING

✻ Very lightly jog on the spot. Here is your opportunity to get into the music! Pump your arms to the rhythm and change the direction you are facing as you jog.

> ### TRAINING TIP
> Spot jogging is a great linking move between exercises. It keeps your heart rate up while you might be considering your next activity.

Quick check

Combine all five moves in this low-impact workout to make a routine that will keep you moving for 20 minutes or so. After 10 minutes, march on the spot and take your pulse to check if you are in your lower target zone.

▶ If you are: keep moving at the same pace.

▶ If your pulse is over the desired figure: slow the moves down slightly.

▶ If your pulse is under the desired figure: put more energy into each move, make the movements larger and maybe even put on faster music to ensure you up the pace a little!

> ### TRAINING TIP
> Adding jumps off two feet – and landing back on two – really ups the work rate. Try spot jogging followed by eight jumps repeated twice to get the heart really pumping.

Walking wonders

One of the best ways to improve cardiovascular fitness without too much planning or effort is walking. Walking can be done anywhere at virtually any time and, if done with a view to working hard, can really contribute to your fitness.

The disadvantage with walking is that it does take time! In order to build a challenging programme, from time to time you may need to do a longer walk that takes 2–3 hours. Don't be put off, however, as this may be a workout you can fit into your schedule on weekends. If you're away somewhere, building a 2–3-hour walk into your schedule is a good way to explore the area while improving fitness at the same time. A walking workout, therefore, is a great tool to have in your fitness tool kit, since you can use it to fit in easily with your busy life – that's the way a good fitness habit should be!

Don't forget to use your pulse check occasionally to see how hard you are working and alter your pace accordingly. With a walking workout, you should find your pulse check shows that you are in the 55–70 per cent heart rate range.

Walking mechanics

When you walk for fitness, stride out with arms swinging by your sides. As each foot steps forward, touch the heel to the ground first, then roll through the foot to the toes. Concentrate on pushing off with your toes to propel yourself into the next step. Don't try to lengthen your stride, rather aim for smaller but quicker steps to up the pace. The faster you move your arms, the faster your legs will go. As you reach a fast pace you will notice your breathing will increase with the effort.

Walking safety

If possible, walk during the day and in places that are well populated. If you do end up walking at twilight or in the dark, make sure you are wearing a white top and ideally some reflective trainers. Carry water to keep yourself well hydrated and consider carrying a mobile phone to call someone if you should need to. The point is to walk a good distance, so get inspired to explore wider areas around where you live. Why not grab a friend and rope them into your walking workouts too?

Your walking programme

If you choose a walking walkout, don't forget to keep to the same structure as other workouts: warm-up, peak activity then cool-down.

✳ To warm up as you begin your walking programme, just get into a slow stride. Don't worry about the speed, the important thing is to loosen up your muscles and find a rhythm.

✳ After 5–10 minutes of warm-up, begin to pump your arms hard and stride out more quickly. Keep breathing regularly and check you can still talk to the person next to you!

✳ During the cool-down phase, slow the pace again and lengthen your stride in order to stretch out the muscles slightly.

✳ Finish the workout with the Express stretch on pages 56–59.

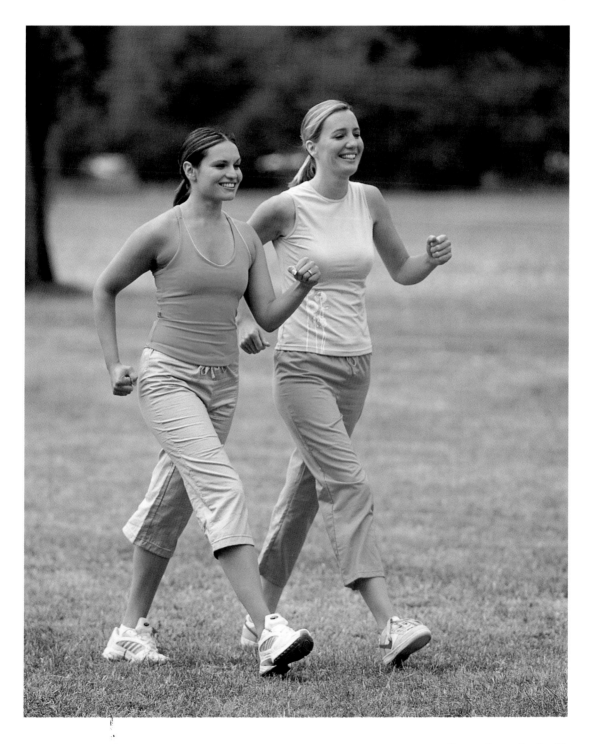

Jogging and running

Like walking, of course, jogging and running are free activities that provide excellent cardio exercise. The following workouts are designed to push your heart rate so that when you check your pulse it is in the higher range: 70–85 per cent.

Jogging mechanics

Pump your arms, just like you do when power-walking, to impel your legs to keep going. And just like walking, be sure that your heel touches the ground first before the rest of your foot.

Many people, when they start to jog, take off too quickly – they race off down the road and then find they have to stop after 100 metres, gasping and spluttering. The key to building a jogging regime is to start slowly. Start barely faster than your walking workout pace and slowly gather speed from there. The body takes a few minutes to shift into cardiovascular mode, so give it time. After 10 minutes or so, if you can keep the pace going, you will probably find you start to settle into a rhythm and the whole jogging process will feel more comfortable.

1 BEGINNER'S JOG

When you're starting out with jogging or have only small amounts of time in your day for a workout, try this simple idea.

✳ Set a stopwatch for 5 minutes.

✳ Leave your home and start jogging. Don't worry about where you are going (as long as it's a safe area) and keep moving (even if it's slowly).

✳ When you've done the 5 minutes, turn around and simply jog back again. This way you'll have done a 10-minute jog and you're back at your house ready to stretch out!

2 PUSH THE PACE

This jog is the same idea as the one above but with one variation: this time you need to get back to your home in 4 minutes, rather than 5! This will push the pace and up your cardiovascular challenge.

3 EXTENDED JOG

Extend your jogging to 10 minutes out and 10 minutes back. As you jog, vary the moves. Try skipping, jogging backwards or side-skipping in 1-minute slots between minutes of jogging.

TRAINING TIPS

Don't forget to check your pulse during the peak of your workout phase.

If you find your pulse is in the 55–70 per cent range, up the pace a little to work yourself slightly harder.

If you find your pulse is in the 70–85 per cent range and you're feeling fine then you can keep the pace as it is.

If you find your pulse is over the 70–85 per cent range, you need to slow things down a little.

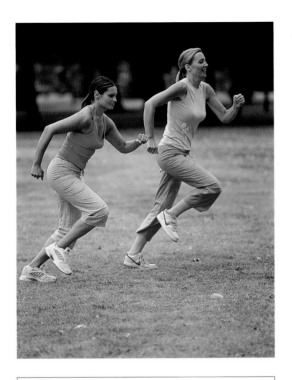

Speedplay

Varying the speed of your running workouts is the key to improving your running fitness. Once you have established a basic running routine of approximately 30 minutes (15 minutes out, 15 minutes back, for example), then you can work on improving the time it takes you.

To do this, start to speed up a small part of your outward run. For example, try sprinting for one minute and then slow back to your normal pace to recover. Try this twice during your run.

Try these other ideas for varying your run:

▶ Run backwards for 50 paces.

▶ Skip sideways for 50 paces, swinging your arms as you go.

▶ Sprint for one minute as fast as you can.

▶ Lift your knees up as high as you can while pumping your arms.

As you begin to incorporate these variations into your run, you will be increasing the intensity and this will start to speed up your overall pace.

TRAINING TIPS

Use this technique to challenge yourself and vary your otherwise steady pace.

If you are having a hard week or have been ill, then leave this session for a week until you feel on top form to attempt it again.

Regular use of this technique will really improve your running times and cardiovascular fitness.

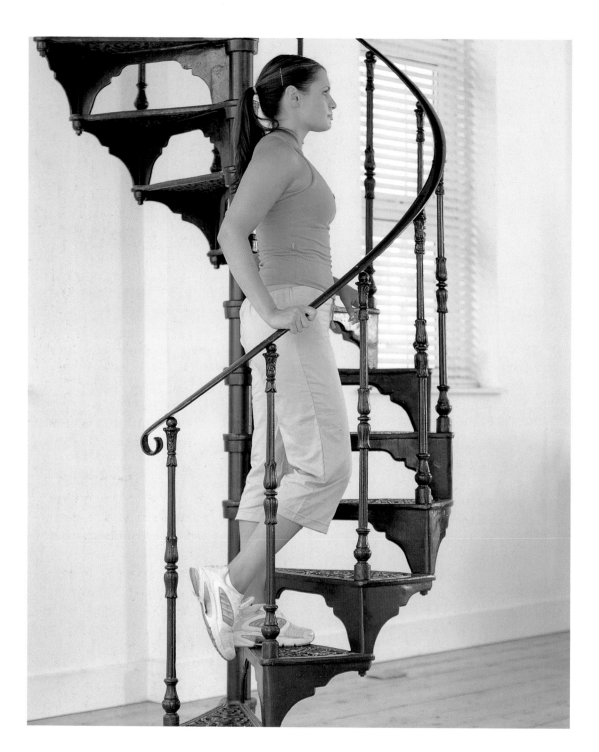

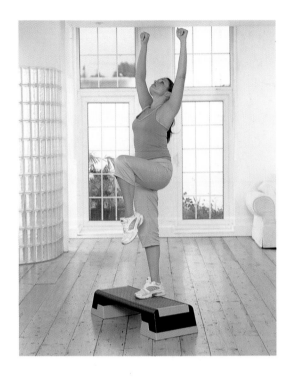

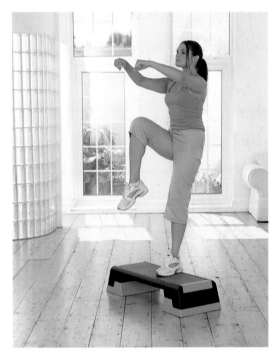

Stair step routine

Why not make use of the stairs in your house for a home workout? They are a great tool for pushing your cardio endurance and for getting the most out of a training session. If you don't have stairs in your home, you have two options: buy a step from a sports shop and adapt the workout to this or hit the park and find some steps you can use out and about in your neighbourhood. Put on some music and work your way through this fun routine.

1 WARM-UP

✳ Start by stepping up and down on just one step. Simply step up and step down, pumping your arms as you go and breathing regularly. Work to the beat of the music and keep it going at the same level of intensity for two minutes.

✳ Now increase the pace so that you begin to step up two steps at a time and back down again: up two, down two. You will notice this is harder work and your breathing will increase accordingly.

✳ Now keep stepping up one step and down one again and then add some different moves, as in the exercises that follow.

2 ARMS OVERHEAD

✳ As you step up, pump your arms over your head. Bring them back down to your sides when you descend.

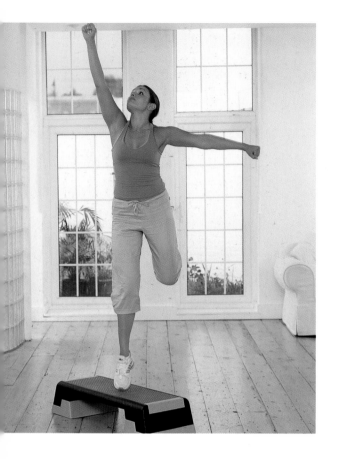

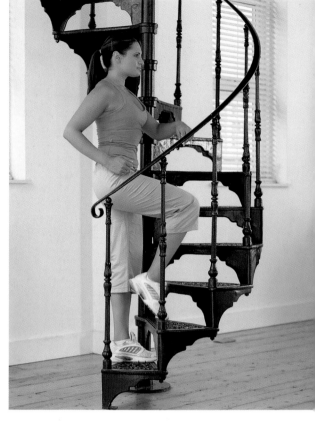

3 ARMS OUT

✳ Step and pump your arms forward as you go. Pretend you are hitting someone in front of you.

4 KNEE HOPS

✳ As you step up one step, bend the non-supporting knee to lift your leg behind. Repeat, alternating legs.

✳ Once you've got the hang of it, add a hop on the supporting leg – this small extra bounce will make you work harder than you think.

✳ Perform the knee hops for 8 or 10 counts, first on one leg, then on the other. Add arm movements to get them stretching and reaching.

5 UPSTAIRS JOG

✳ If you're working on a stairwell, jog up three stairs and jog backwards down again. Repeat 10 times.

✳ Start to challenge your endurance with this move: jump up on to the first step and step back down. Repeat 20 times.

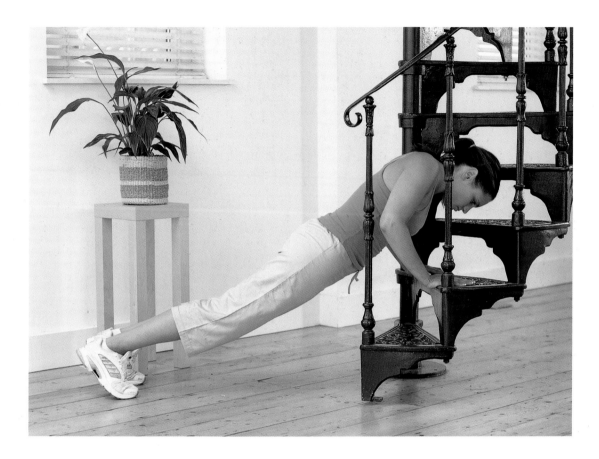

6 STEP PUSH-UPS

✻ Stand at the bottom of a stairwell. Lean forward and place your hands on the third or fourth step – or one that you can reach comfortably. Perform 10 push-ups before returning to the basic step-up-step-down routine.

7 STAIR INTERVALS

✻ Now you can use the full extent of your stairwell as your goal is to jog carefully all the way up to the top and back down again.

✻ When you reach the top of the stairs, perform five knee hops.

✻ Next, jog back down again. Repeat this sequence five times.

✻ To finish this routine, stand at the bottom of the stairwell with your back to the stairs. Place your hands on the third step up – or one that you can reach comfortably. Perform 10 triceps dips (see page 121).

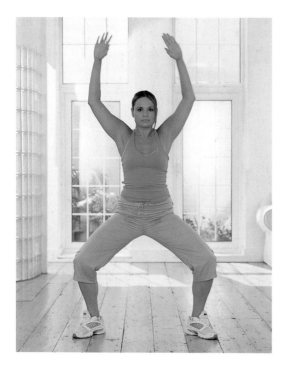

Circuit workout

Another great way to get an aerobic workout is to create a circuit system. The idea behind circuits is to perform a variety of exercises for a set amount of time, working different parts of the body, in order to challenge your endurance. Because you move quickly from one station to another, you also keep your heart rate up and, if planned carefully, you can keep the whole workout at the target aerobic level (see page 26 for more on heart rates).

So get creative and make your own mini stations in your home. You can make good use of some of your furniture as well as any other fitness equipment you have to build a fun workout.

The circuit template

✶ Start with a warm-up routine of 5–10 minutes (see chapter 3 for ideas for warm-up moves).

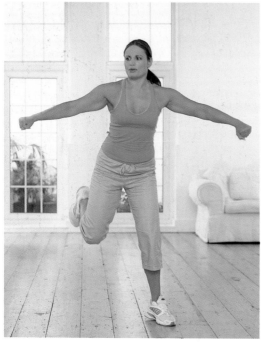

✶ Now work your way around each circuit station. You should ideally set yourself four or five different station activities. Give yourself 2 minutes on each station to work through the move as cleanly and carefully as you can. Your aim is to perform as many repetitions of that move as you can in the 2 minutes without compromising on technique.

✶ When you have finished at one station, take a 1-minute interval. During this time, jog on the spot, skip side to side or just keep moving in order to keep your heart rate up. If you have been working hard enough during the previous station, you should need this minute to recover your breath and prepare yourself mentally for the next station.

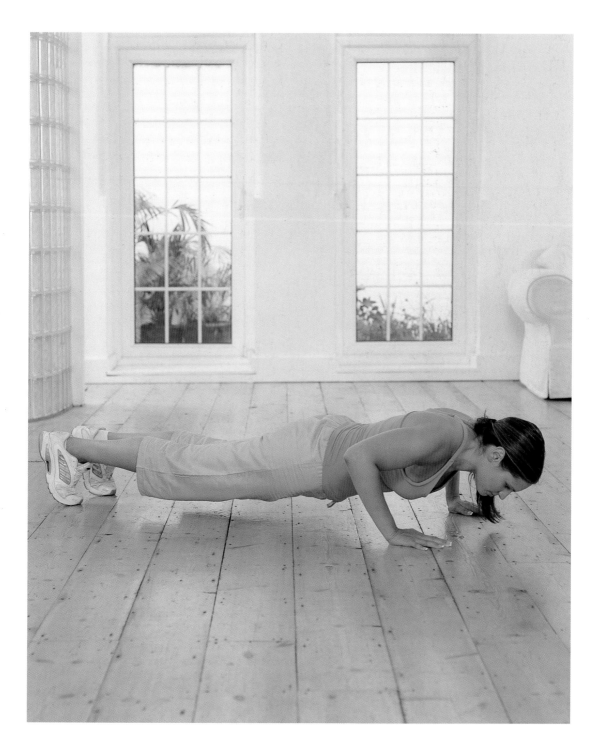

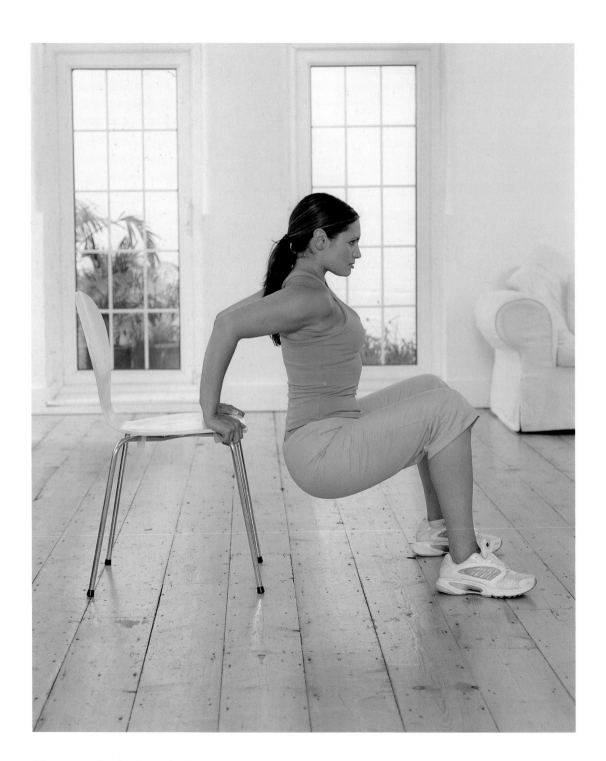

Station ideas

The stations you set up in your home are limited only by your imagination. Just try something new each time you do a circuit workout – keeping things different and interesting means you're more likely to keep up an exercise regime. Here are some simple ideas for which you need no special equipment:

▶ Star jumps: start with your feet together and arms by your sides. Jump both feet apart sideways with arms straight out to the sides at the same time, to form a star shape. Jump back in. Repeat.

▶ Push-ups: perform full push-ups on the floor.

▶ Tricep dips: sit on the edge of a sofa or other sturdy chair. Place your hands under your bottom on the edge of the seat. Inch your bottom off the seat and bend your legs. Now lower your body towards the floor by bending your arms as you dip, then straightening your arms to lift back up.

▶ Fast jog: jog on the spot as quickly as you possibly can, lifting your knees right up and pumping your arms.

▶ Spotty dogs: this is a silly move with a silly name, but good fun! Jump with the right foot forward and the left foot behind to form a walking position. Take the right arm forward to match the right leg and the left arm back to match the left leg. (This goes against your natural tendency to use opposite arms and legs.) Bounce on your feet and then switch arms and legs to the other direction in one quick jump. Continue to bounce back and forward, rolling through the feet as you land.

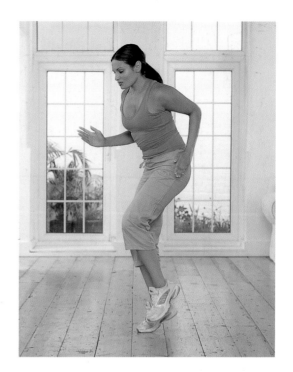

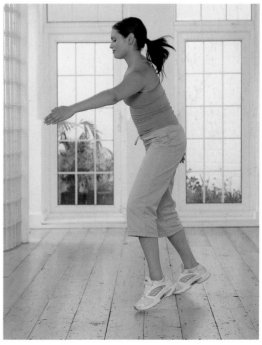

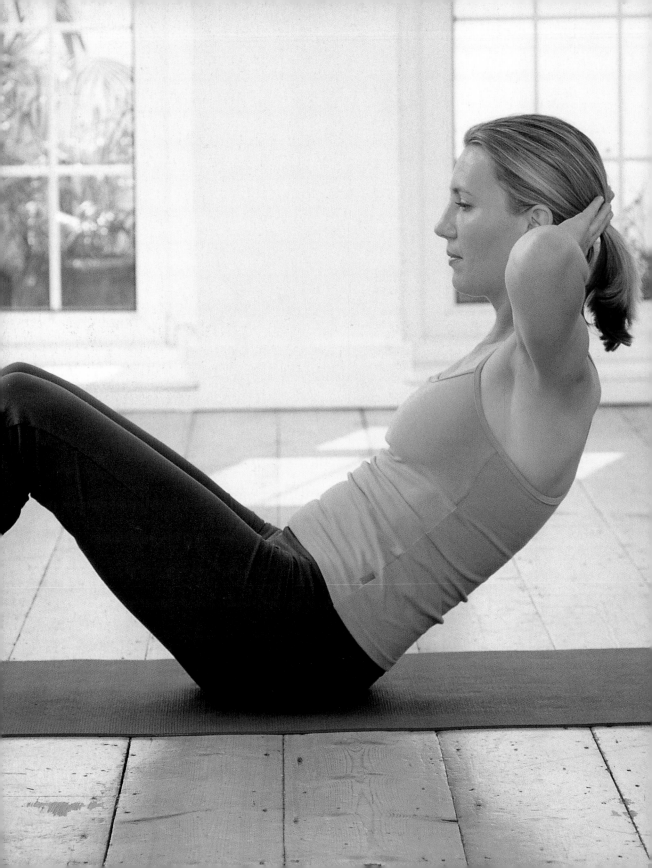

chapter 5

abs and back

This section focuses on spot training the abdominal area. While spot training is not effective on its own, as part of a balanced programme it can make a big difference to the focus muscle area. The stomach area, where the abdominal muscles lie, is often neglected. Lax muscles can lead not only to a flabby stomach but back problems. Happily, a little core strengthening in this area can combat back problems and improve the shape of your torso almost immediately.

Posture perfecter

Before you embark on a serious abs workout for the first time – or for the first time in a long while – stop to remind yourself of some good posture habits. Learning how to lie and stand properly, as well as engaging the deep abdominal muscles that run horizontally across the stomach and help support the whole torso area, will make a huge difference to your posture and the tone of your stomach area. Practise the two basic pelvic postures that follow until they become instinctive. Practise them enough times that each time you stand up, you naturally adopt the aligned, correct posture you've learned here.

1 PRONE PELVIC TILT

* Lie on your back with your knees bent and feet flat on the floor. Rest your head and arms on the floor.

* Try to push your lower back into the floor as much as you can. Notice the feeling when you do this; what happens to the abdominal muscles? You should feel them tightening. You should also feel your hip bones tip upwards slightly as the deep and superficial abdominal muscles contract.

* Release the contraction and allow your lower back to come off the floor slightly. Notice the relaxed mode of the abdominals.

* Perform the pelvic tilt lying on the floor eight times. The purpose of this exercise is not only to tone the abdominals but to make you aware of the posture you should be striving for when standing.

2 STANDING PELVIC CORRECTION

* Come to a standing position with your back very near a flat wall. Now perform the same pelvic tilt as in the previous move. Start with your stomach relaxed and your hands on your hips.

* Push your lower back towards the wall and tilt your hips upwards by pushing down on your thumbs and pulling up with your fingers. Again, note the tension across your stomach. By tilting the pelvis just slightly, you are tightening the transverse muscles.

* Now keep the tension in the stomach but relax your arms by your side and pull your shoulders back. From here you need to adjust your position slightly. Don't hold yourself too stiffly – try to relax into it. Make sure your weight is equally divided between the heels and balls of your feet. Lift the top of your head towards the ceiling – and try to feel a lifting through the whole body.

* Practise this standing posture, holding for one minute, two or three times. Alternate with the prone pelvic tilt.

TRAINING TIP

If you aim to adopt this posture whenever you stand for any length of time, you will be getting into a very good habit of keeping your spine lengthened and your stomach muscles working. It is also a painless and easy way to keep your stomach toned.

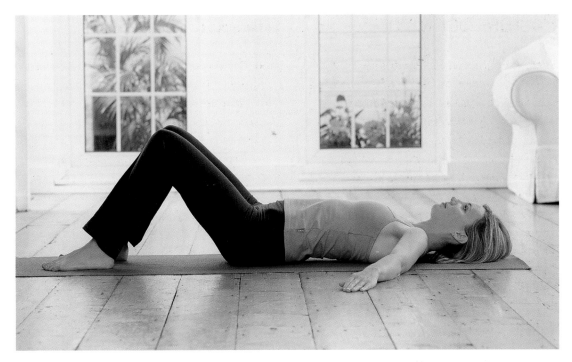

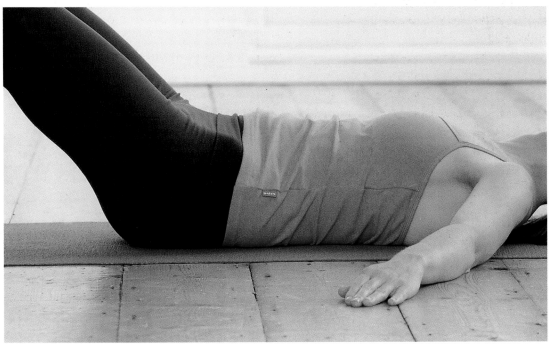

Express abdominal workout

Once you have mastered the basics on the previous pages, move on to this quick but effective abs workout. This should take 10 minutes or so. If you want to make it longer, simply repeat the workout or combine it with one of the others in this chapter to form a 20-minute block.

This express routine includes an exercise to strengthen the back and stretch out the torso for a complete rehab of the abs!

1 PELVIC TILT AND LIFT

✳ Lie on your back with your knees bent and your feet flat on the floor. Rest your arms by your sides.

✳ Begin by tilting your pelvis and pressing your lower back into the floor, just like in the prone pelvic tilt (page 84).

✳ Continue the movement by pushing down on your feet and lifting your lower back and bottom off the floor. Press your hips high into the air while pulling in on your stomach. Hold for 10 seconds, then release and come back down.

✳ Repeat eight to ten times. Rest briefly and do another set of eight to ten.

TRAINING TIPS
As you press the hips upwards, think about pulling your stomach towards your spine to really flatten it.

As you lower your back down again, try to curve your spine so that it feels as though each individual vertebra was being placed down on the floor one by one. This will help avoid injury.

Building a sixpack

The more abdominal crunches you do, the more muscular your stomach will become. If you are really intent on building a 'washboard stomach', then you need to perform at least 100–200 ab curls a day.

Try putting together five different moves from this chapter, performing 20 of each. You will easily make up the 100 moves you need. Stick at this for two weeks and you will notice a real difference!

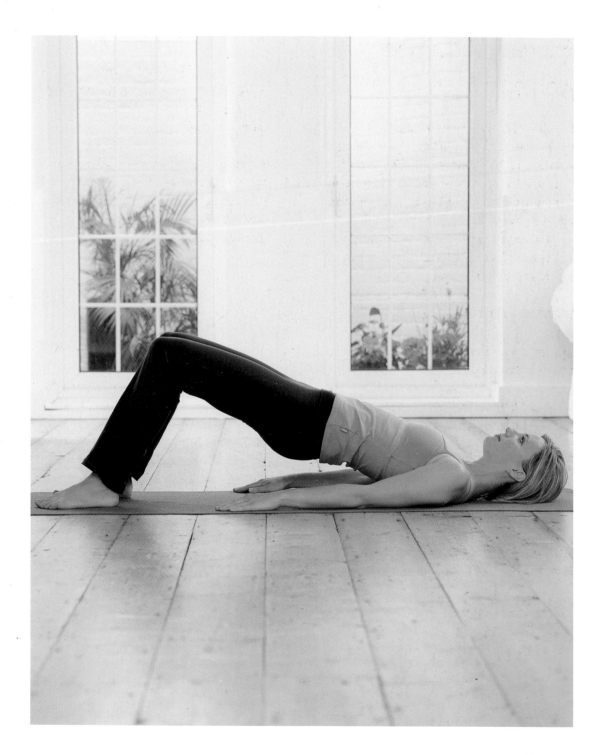

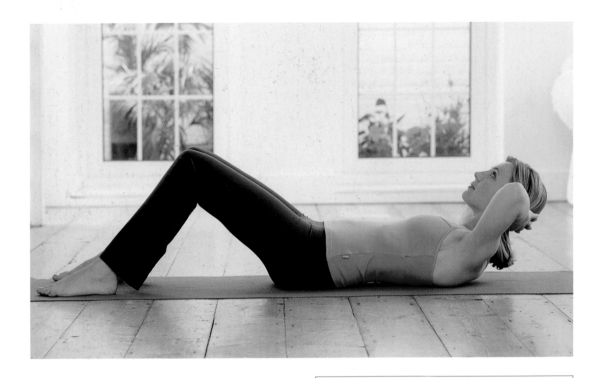

2 STOMACH CURL

✳ Lie on your back with your knees bent and your hands behind your head.

✳ Slowly push your head and shoulders off the ground, towards the ceiling, exhaling as you come up. Hold for a few seconds.

✳ Lower your head and shoulders back to the ground in a slow, controlled manner.

TRAINING TIP

Many people rush through their abdominal workout without checking that they are flattening as well as working the muscles. To do this you need to slow the movement down and concentrate on the flattening movement during each muscle contraction. Once you have checked that your technique is correct, proceed with the crunches, looking up to the ceiling as you pull upwards.

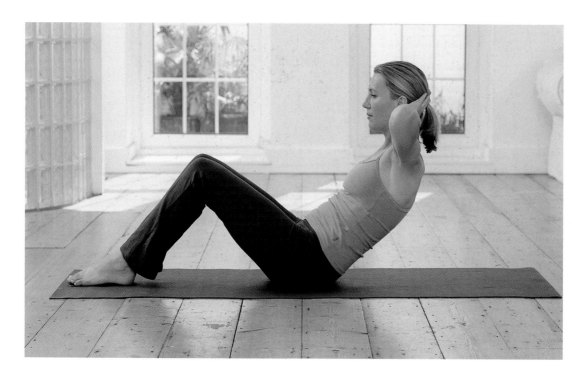

3 ADVANCED SIT-UPS

Advanced sit-ups are the old-school sit-ups many of us were taught as children. They fell out of favour because they were considered potentially dangerous for the back. However, done carefully, these sit-ups can be very useful in an overall abs routine.

The important thing to remember is that these sit-ups should be done only when your stomach is quite strong and when there is no discomfort in your back.

✳ Lie on your back with knees bent and feet pressed into the floor. Place your hands behind your head.

✳ Curl your head and shoulders slowly off the floor and continue to peel your back off the floor until you are sitting upright.

✳ Slowly lower your back down to the floor. Repeat eight times, carefully coming up and down.

TRAINING TIP

Remember that the most important part of this move is to keep the back curving like a piece of rubber hose. The minute you feel your back start to lift in one piece like a stiff board, then you know your stomach muscles are wimping out! So rest for a moment and then attempt to begin again.

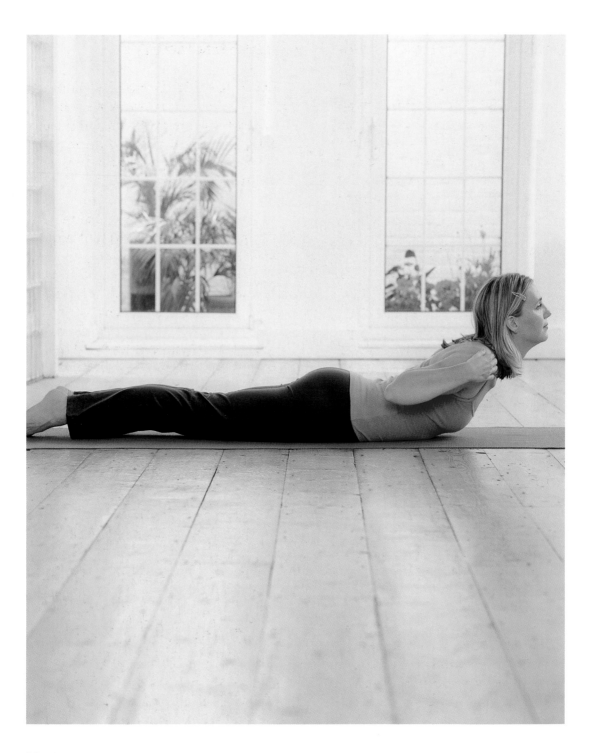

Back work

Once you have done some work on your abdominals, it is always wise to complement this with work on the back muscles. Working opposing sets of muscles in the same workout is good practice as it helps keep you balanced. While your abs have been contracted and working hard from the previous exercises, they will feel a stretch when you work your back muscles.

4 HYPEREXTENSION

✳ Lie on your front with your legs straight and hands tucked under your shoulders.

✳ Tighten your buttocks and legs and lift your head and chest off the floor, keeping your hands on your shoulders.

✳ Arch up as high as is comfortable before slowly releasing back down.

✳ Repeat this move eight to ten times.

TRAINING TIPS
As you get stronger you can take your arms out above your head to increase the load of the lift.

This move strengthens the muscles that run alongside the spine. These muscles help keep your back safe and strong. Strong abs will support your back too.

---

5 ABS AND BACK STRETCH

Finish off your express abs workout with a stretch. When you work any muscles repetitively and consistently it is good practice to return them to their original length again with a good stretch. Generally, stretch routines neglect the stomach area, so remember this one!

✳ Lie on your front with your legs straight and place your hands directly underneath your shoulders.

✳ Push back on your hands to lift your head and chest off the floor, arching your back.

✳ Hold this position as you breathe naturally, and lower when you are ready.

✳ Repeat several times. You will feel a glorious stretch across the front of your stomach as well as an opening out of the chest.

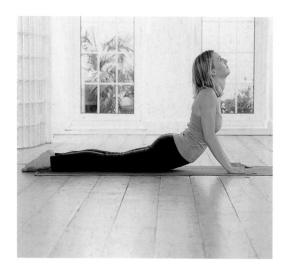

Extended abdominal workout

When you have more than 10 minutes in your day for abs work, you can start to include some more advanced exercises in your programme.

Remember that there are three sets of abdominal muscles: the rectus abdominus (the 'sixpack' muscles), the transverse muscles and the external and internal obliques (see page 16). To get your stomach as strong as possible, you need to do exercises that keep all these sets of muscles strong. The reverse curl, below, will tone your rectus abdominus and the twisting crunch, opposite, works both the oblique and the rectus. In the yoga abs moves (pages 94–95), you will focus more on the transverse mucles. Learn and perfect these exercises for a rock-hard abdomen!

REVERSE CURL

✷ Lie on your back and rest your arms by your sides. Cross your legs together at the ankles in the air.

✷ Lift your hips and lower back off the floor by squeezing on your abdominals tightly. This move is harder than it looks, so take a few moments to attempt the lift and then relax. When you first attempt this move you may need to swing your legs slightly to help you with the motion of lifting your hips off the floor. You might also feel the need to press down with your hands on the floor to facilitate the lifting. As you get stronger you will need to do this less and less.

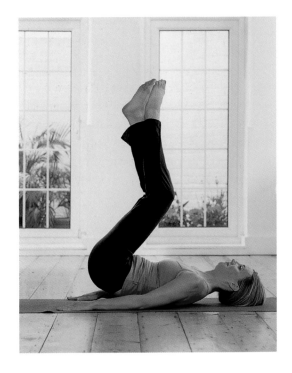

✷ Repeat this move 10 times. Recover for 30 seconds, then do another 10.

> **TRAINING TIP**
> As you progress with this move, think about contracting your abdominals and lifting your legs upwards towards the ceiling rather than in towards your torso. This means you are doing more work with the abdominals!

2 TWISTING CRUNCH

This move involves a twisting action that tones the oblique muscles of the abdominal wall, which run in a V shape along your sides. Keeping the oblique muscles in great shape ensures all your twisting and leaning movements are strong and safe.

✳ Lie on your back on the floor with your legs crossed at the ankles in the air. Place your hands behind your head and actively rest your head back into your hands.

✳ Lift up your head and shoulders, twist and press your right elbow towards your left knee.

✳ Lower back down slowly.

✳ Lift up again to press your left elbow towards your right knee, and lower.

✳ Keep lifting and twisting alternately on each side. Repeat 20 times, rest for 30 seconds, then do another set of 20.

3 DOUBLE CRUNCH

This is an endurance move that really challenges your abdominal strength.

✳ Lie on your back on the floor with your hands behind your head and feet flat on the floor.

✳ Lift your upper body off the floor; at the same time aim to lift your lower back off the floor. Exhale as you contract your muscles. Your knees should be bent and pulling in towards your face. In this

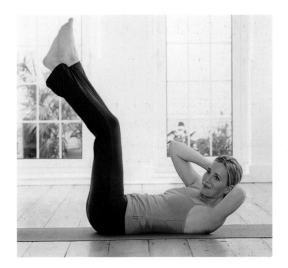

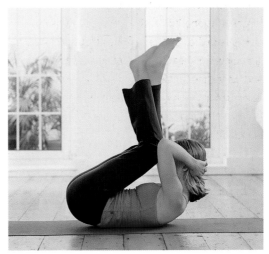

way you are performing a crunch from the top of the body and bottom. Your middle back should be the only part of the body left on the floor.

✳ Release and lower your upper and lower body back down to the floor.

✳ Repeat 20 times, recover for 30 seconds, then do another set of 20.

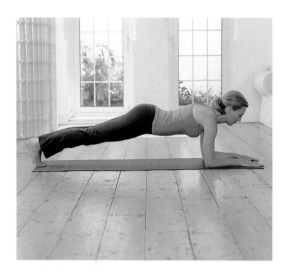

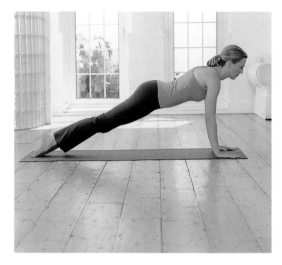

Yoga abs

Yoga postures work the stomach area in different ways. A lot of the positions in yoga utilise the isometric method of training, where muscles are contracted and held for a period of time but are not moving.

Note that moves performed in this way can raise the blood pressure so they should be performed with caution.

BEGINNER PLANK POSE

✳ Rest your body on your lower arms and knees with your toes tucked under your ankles.

✳ Push up on to your feet and straighten your legs so that your body weight is on your forearms and feet. In order to hold this position you are contracting the whole abdominal section in an isometric way. Keep your whole body as flat and straight as possible – exactly like a plank of wood!

✳ Hold the plank position as solidly as you can for up to 30 seconds. Release down on to your knees to recover and repeat.

> **TRAINING TIP**
> With this move it is not the repetition of the exercise that is important but the holding of the position. Resist the urge to give up!

INTERMEDIATE PLANK POSE

✳ This time, start on your hands and knees and rest the tops of your feet on the floor.

✳ Lift your knees up off the floor and rest your body weight on the tops of your feet and your hands. To maintain this position you will have to lift and hold your whole torso in tension.

6 THE BOAT POSE

This position really works the abdominals and the hip muscles. It takes some practice to be able to achieve, but is well worth it once you've got the hang of it.

✳ Sit on your bottom with your knees bent and hands clasped under your knees.

✳ Rock back slightly so that your feet come off the floor.

✳ Release your hands and stretch your arms straight in line with your legs.

✳ If you feel balanced, straighten your legs. If you achieve this you will be in a V shape.

✳ Hold this position for five breaths and then release, bringing your legs slowly down.

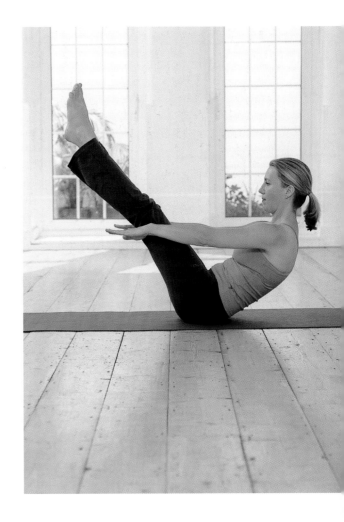

TRAINING TIPS

If you are unable to extend your legs to begin with, don't worry. Keep your knees lifted and your legs bent and maintain this position – it will still tone your stomach.

Keep your shoulders pressed down towards the floor and keep breathing regularly as you hold this position.

Core conditioning

Pilates is a superb body-conditioning regime. As discussed in chapter 1, it began with the work of Joseph Pilates, who developed programmes that were then further influenced by the principles of the Laban dance technique. Pilates eventually set up a studio in New York that attracted elite dancers and other sports people of America, where he further honed his techniques.

One of the major principles of Pilates is its emphasis on strengthening the area around the solar plexus – the centre of the body from which, as dancers know, all other movement radiates. The following three exercises give you a taste of what is involved if you haven't already tried Pilates.

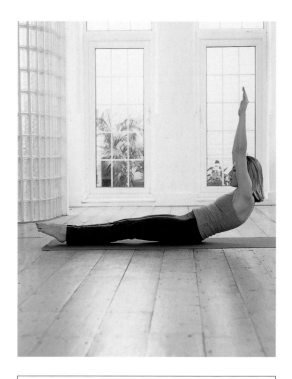

7 THE ROLL-UP

✳ Lie on your back on the floor with your arms straight above your head. Extend your feet away from you and press your shoulders down.

✳ As you breathe in, slowly lift your arms up toward the ceiling.

✳ Now begin to breathe out as you peel your upper body and spine slowly off the floor.

✳ Keep the movement flowing as you breathe in again and lay your torso down over your legs.

✳ Finally, breathing out, roll slowly down to the floor again, and repeat.

TRAINING TIPS

Focus on using your abdominals – they should be taut but not scrunched up. The strengthening comes from performing this move in a slow, controlled manner.

Don't forget to stretch out your stomach muscles after working them hard in an exercise such as this. Use the abs and back stretch on page 91.

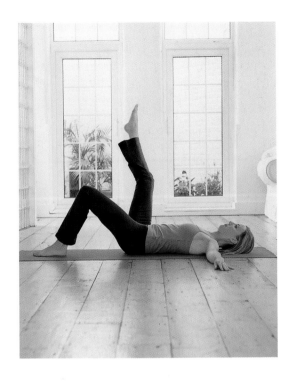

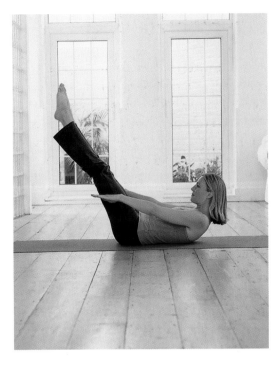

8 ONE-LEG CIRCLE

✳ Lie on your back with your knees bent and feet flat on the floor. Relax your arms on the floor straight out to the side.

✳ Contract your abdominals and lift one leg to the ceiling. Keep your back pushed close to the floor. Allow the knee to bend slightly and slowly circle the leg first one way and then the other. Be aware of the tension in your lower abdominal area so that you can start to appreciate the work done by your abs to control the leg. Repeat five times with each leg.

9 THE HUNDRED

✳ Lie on your back with your hands by your sides. Point your toes, extending your legs and press your shoulders down to the floor.

✳ Lift your legs until they are at a 45-degree angle from the floor and your head and chest are lifted.

✳ Stretch your arms out towards your knees.

✳ Now lift and lower your arms, as if pumping to keep the abdominals tight, all the while breathing in and out in rhythm. Pump your arms 30 times before releasing and lowering. Recover for 30 seconds and repeat.

Working the waist

When you bend over to one side or twist around behind you to see over your shoulder, you are using the muscles of the abdominals that wrap around the sides and front of your torso. If you use these muscles regularly and work on twisting and bending moves, you will find your waist tightening and toning and gaining much more flexibility. The following yoga postures are excellent moves for working the waist area.

10 TRIANGLE POSE

✳ Stand with your feet wide apart.

✳ Turn your right foot out 90 degrees and keep your left foot pointing straight ahead.

✳ Reach both arms out straight to the sides.

✳ Flex your right thigh and slowly lean over to the right, extending from the waist and reaching towards the floor. Keep your legs straight at all times. Your arms, shoulders and hips should be aligned in a vertical plane.

✳ If you can, link your fingers under your right big toe and hold while you breathe five controlled breaths.

✳ While holding this posture, try to push your left shoulder forwards and your right shoulder back to the vertical. Repeat on the left side.

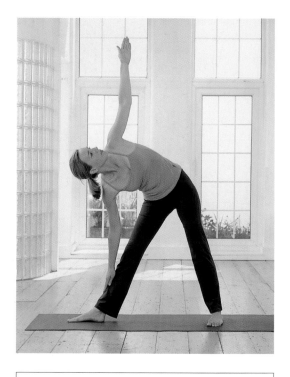

TRAINING TIP

If you can't reach to hook your fingers under your toes, simply place your hand on your shin.

---

11 GATE POSE

✳ Start by kneeling on both knees with your back straight up tall.

✳ Take your right leg out to the side at a 90-degree angle, keeping it straight.

✳ Extend your right foot and turn it outwards so that you can press your toes toward the ground.

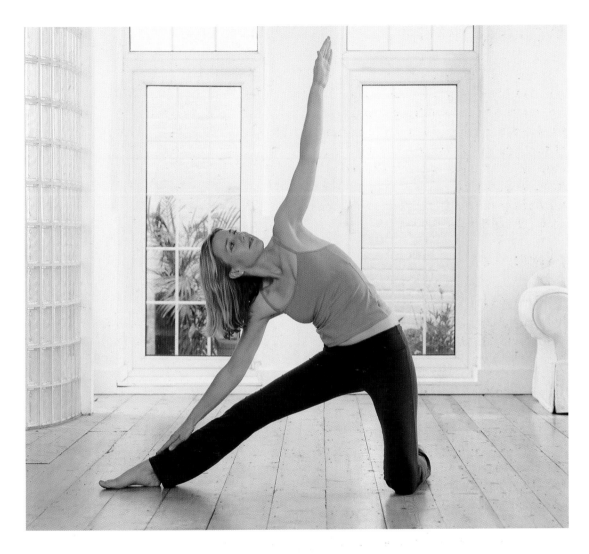

✳ Extend both arms straight out to the sides.

✳ Reach with your torso and arms over to the right side. Tip your upper body, lift your left arm up straight into the air as you reach your right arm straight down towards your right shin. Look up to your left hand. As you lean into the bend, you will feel a deep stretch on your left side.

✳ If you can, place your right hand on your right shin. Hold this position for five breaths.

✳ Lift up slowly, to bring yourself back to centre. As you lift up, focus on using the muscles on the left side of the torso.

✳ Perform this move twice on each side.

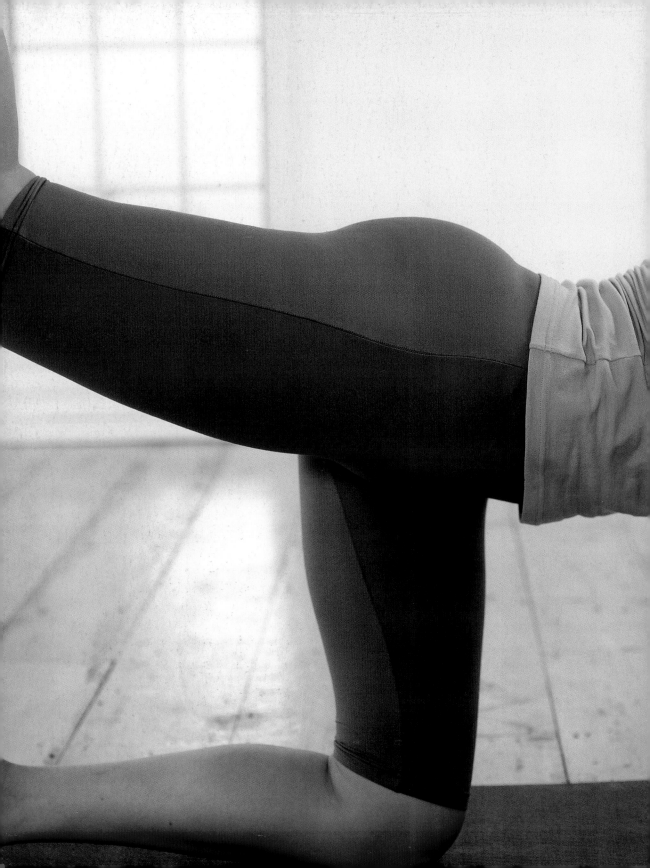

chapter 6
hips, thighs and bum

This section focuses on spot training the hips, thighs and bum.
Many women (and some men) find this is the area where they
tend to collect fat. But don't despair! With regular targeted work
you will notice a real difference. While spot training the muscle
area alone is not enough, when you couple this with targeted
cardiovascular training you really do give yourself the best chance
of gaining toned hips and thighs with less cellulite and more shape.

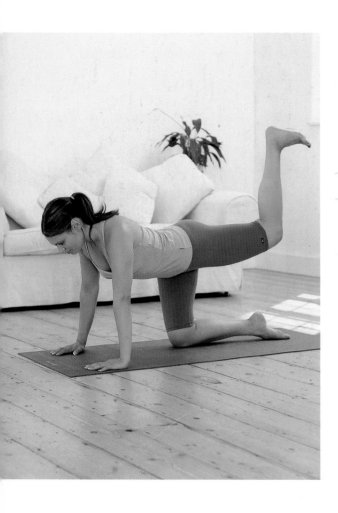

Working the buttocks

Much of the work for the buttocks can be done on all fours. Grab a yoga mat or kneel on a rug, put on your favourite smooth tunes, and work that bottom area for a good 10–20 minutes.

1 REAR-LEG RAISES

✳ On your hands and knees, position your weight equally between all fours.

✳ Contract your abdominals and ensure your back is as straight as a table top.

✳ Lift one leg behind you and upwards. The leg should be bent and the sole of your foot should be facing the ceiling.

✳ Pulse the leg up and down very gently, moving just a couple of centimetres at a time. Perform 20 pulses then lower the leg to the floor.

✳ Repeat with the other leg, then follow with another set of 20 pulses on each leg.

> ### TRAINING TIP
> This move works the buttocks very hard. If you can't feel your buttock muscles working, make sure your leg is lifted up high enough.

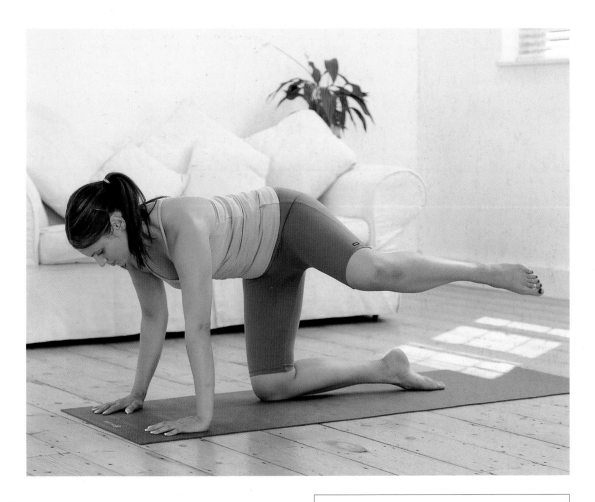

2 SIDE-LEG RAISES

✳ This exercise starts in the same position as the rear-leg raise. Begin on all fours, but this time lift one leg out to the side with a bent knee. Your leg should be at right angles to your body, and the knee and ankle should be parallel with the ground.

✳ Now pulse the leg up and down 20 times.

✳ Lower and repeat with the other leg. Follow with another set of 20 pulses on each leg.

TRAINING TIP

As you perform this exercise you may feel some tiredness in the lifting thigh. If you feel a burning sensation, this is the lactic acid building up in the muscle as it runs out of energy. If this occurs, lower the leg briefly in order to recover and then continue.

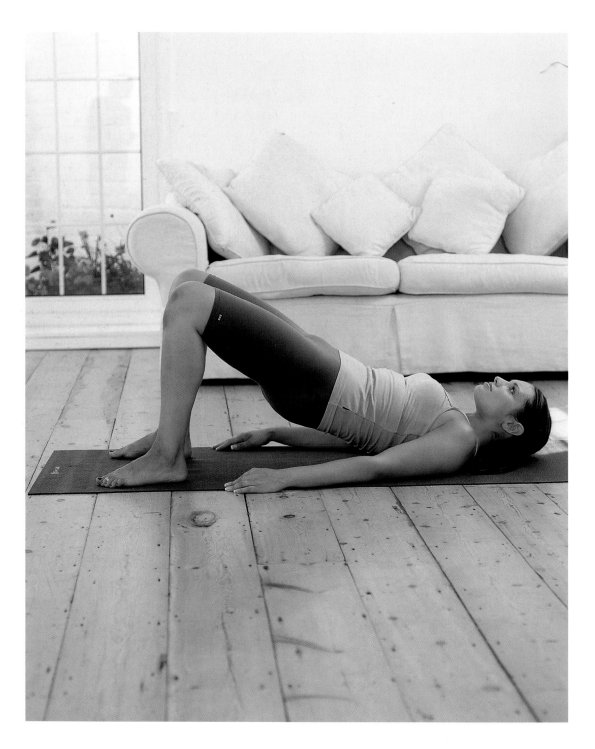

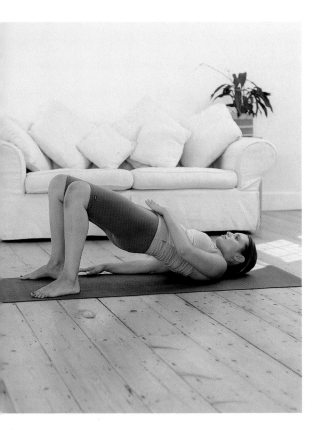

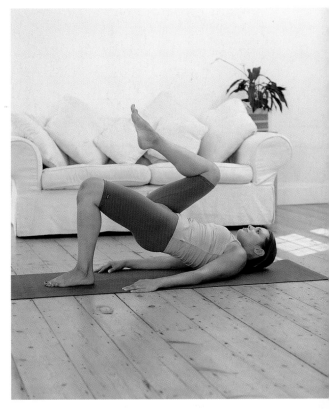

3 BUTTOCK SQUEEZES

✻ Lie on your back with your knees bent and feet on the floor. Rest your hands by your sides.

✻ First, perform the prone pelvic tilt (see page 84) and then lift your hips high into the air.

✻ As you reach the top of the lift, squeeze your buttock muscles as tightly as possible then slowly lower your hips back down to the floor.

✻ Repeat, hold and pulse first for 5 seconds, then 10, then 30.

TRAINING TIP

Once you've mastered the buttock squeezes try some variations. Open and squeeze closed your legs while your pelvis is in the air, squeezing the buttocks as you close your legs. Alternatively, to really up the load, try carefully lifting one foot off the floor while your hips are in the air, bringing the knee in towards the body, and pulsing the hips upwards as before.

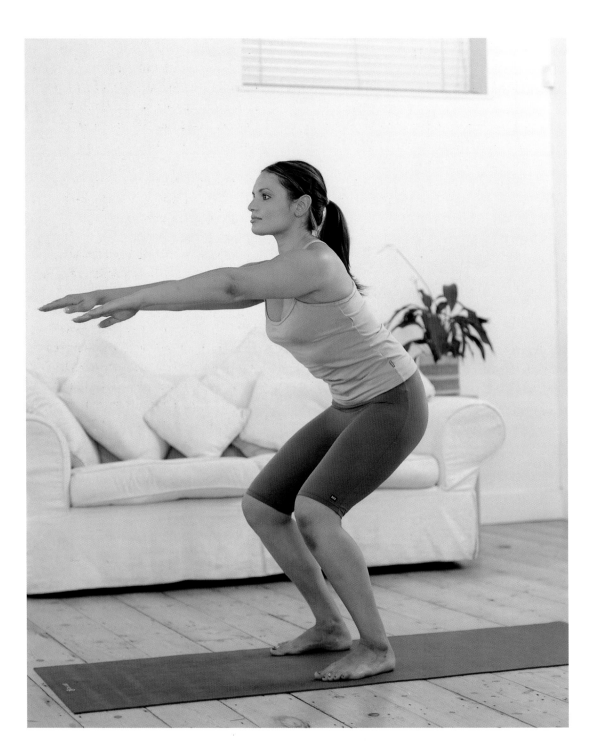

Working the hips and thighs

There are some essential moves when it comes to training the hips and thighs. These moves target all the major muscles of these areas and work them extremely effectively. There's no need for added weights – your body weight is everything you need to work these muscle groups.

1 THE SQUAT

✳ Stand with your feet hip-width apart and with your arms by your sides.

✳ Push your bottom out behind you and slowly lower your body down, as if you were about to sit down on a chair.

✳ Lower your bottom until your thighs are nearly parallel with the floor.

✳ Reach your arms out in front of you for balance.

✳ Hold for three breaths and then press through your legs to come to a full standing position again.

✳ Repeat 10 times, recover for 30 seconds, then perform another set of 10.

TRAINING TIPS

This is one of those moves that appears simple but is difficult to get right. Use a mirror, if possible, to check you are performing it correctly.

Make sure your bottom is sticking out behind you, so that your weight is over your heels as you lower down.

Your hips up to your shoulders should be in a straight line, with your abdominals tight and pelvic floor pulled up.

Whenever you go to lift anything heavy, adopt the squat position to make sure you are doing it safely. If you lower yourself this way, grasp what you need to pick up and then press through the legs to lift, you will not only be toning your thighs but protecting your back as well.

2 THE LUNGE

✳ Start standing, with your weight equally divided between your feet.

✳ Take one leg behind you so that the back foot has just the toes touching the floor. Contract the stomach muscles and tilt your hips under slightly so that you feel a slight stretch along the front of the right side of your hip.

✳ Bend both legs so that your hips drop directly towards the floor. You should feel your thighs working hard – particularly the thigh of the back leg.

✳ Press down with your legs to straighten your body up again.

✳ Repeat 20 times then swap legs for another set of 20.

TRAINING TIP

It is very important to check that, as you bend, you do not press your front knee too far forward over your foot. The knee should stay in line with your foot as you bend, otherwise you will be putting too much pressure on it.

---

3 THIGH LIFTS

✳ Sit upright on a chair.

✳ Lift up through the body, feeling energy pressing out of the top of the head as you straighten the spine.

✳ Flex one foot by pulling the top of the foot upwards so that the toe is lifted and the Achilles is stretched.

✳ Now simply lift that leg until it is straight out in front of you, parallel with the floor.

✳ Slowly release it back down again.

✳ Lift and lower the leg while breathing regularly.

✳ Perform 30 lifts on each leg, recover and repeat the sets of 30.

TRAINING TIP

As you straighten the leg, you are focusing on the quadriceps muscles at the top of the thigh (see page 16).

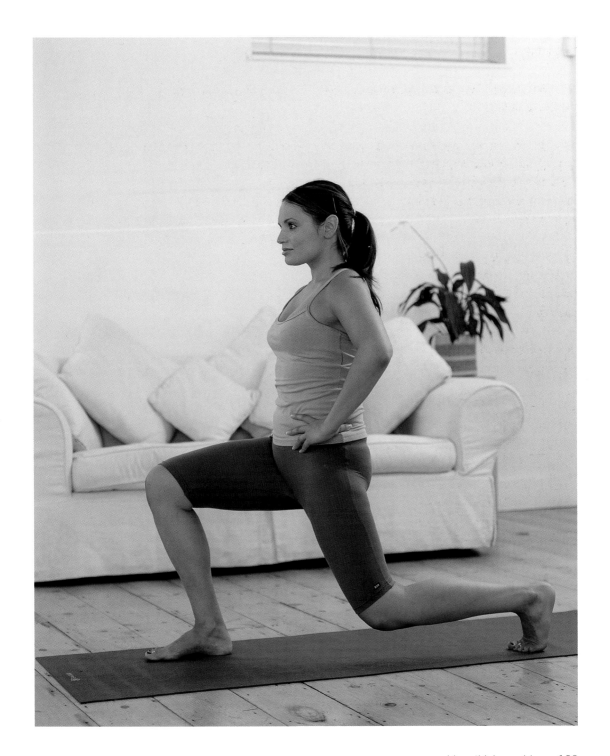

Yoga bum

Several yoga postures require some serious stamina from the buttocks! Holding the poses as you count your breaths tones and sculpts the muscles very effectively. So perform these sequences regularly to develop perfect peaches!

1 WARRIOR POSE

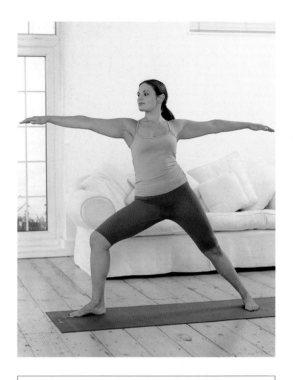

✳ Start this move from the downward-dog position (see page 53). Alternatively, begin on all fours and then lift your knees off the floor.

✳ Bring your right leg forward, bend your right knee and stretch your left leg straight out behind you. Your front foot should be facing forwards and the back foot should turn out at a 45-degree angle.

✳ Lift your body up and square your hips by pulling your right buttock back and pressing your left hip forwards.

✳ Tuck your tail in tightly – this requires further work from the buttocks and ensures the front knee is directly over the front foot.

✳ Now reach up with your arms straight, pressing your palms firmly together. Look up at your hands.

✳ Hold this position for five breaths.

✳ Push your front leg straight to come into a balanced mid position, then swap legs and repeat on the other side.

> ### TRAINING TIP
> When you perform this move, press the outside of the back foot down into the floor and press the supporting knee outwards. Doing this ensures you tone your inner thighs as well as your buttocks. Because they work more than one muscle group at a time, yoga exercises are often called 'combination moves'.

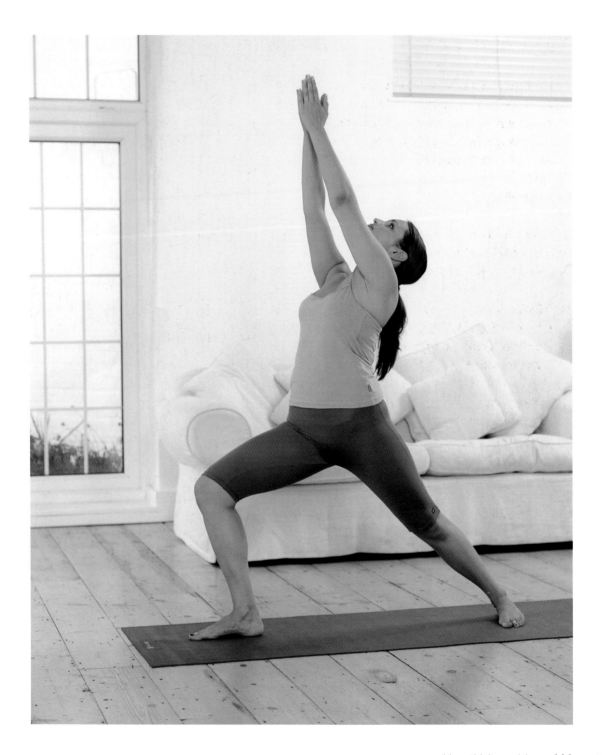

2 FIERCE POSTURE

* Stand with your legs pressed together.

* Begin to sit downwards, sinking into your heels and thighs. Tuck your tailbone in.

* Raise your arms out to the sides and bring them together above your head.

* Press your shoulders down and press your palms together as you reach upwards with the upper body and downwards with the bottom.

* Hold for five breaths. You should notice the work going on in your buttocks and legs.

* Push down through your legs to straighten out of this position.

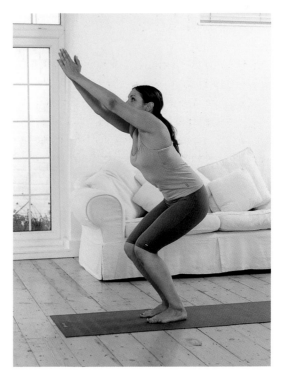

3 PREPARATION FOR SEATED BACK ARCH

This position stretches the front of the legs as well as asking for a lot of work from the buttocks.

* Lie on your back on the floor with your top half resting on your elbows, forearms flat on the floor.

* Push down through your legs to lift your bottom off the floor and lift your hips as high as you can. Squeeze your buttocks to help lift your hips higher.

* Hold this position for two breaths and release back down. Repeat twice.

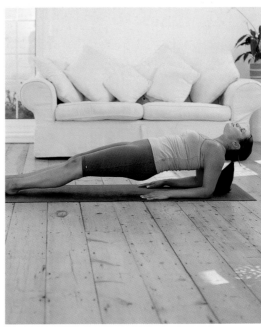

Power thighs

The following four exercises tighten and firm the thighs to give you shape as well as strength. Jumping and lifting your legs not only work your quadriceps at the front of your thighs but shape the sides and backs of your legs as the muscles support your entire body weight while you balance.

1 PLIÉ

❉ Stand with your feet wide apart. Turn out your feet at 45-degree angles.

❉ Place your hands on your hips.

❉ Bend your knees slowly, dropping your bottom directly between your hips as you lower. Keep your bottom tucked in. Your knees should be pointing directly over your toes. Press back upwards in a similar way.

❉ Keep breathing regularly as you slowly bend down through the plié and up again. Repeat 10 to 12 times.

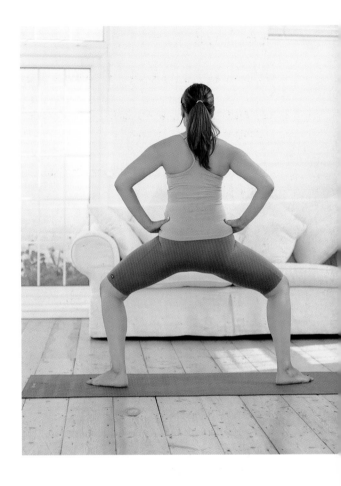

TRAINING TIP
Be careful not to turn out your feet from the ankle. Instead, use the muscles at the back of your legs to turn your legs out-wards and to maintain control. This is the kind of exercise that gives ballet dancers such shapely pins.

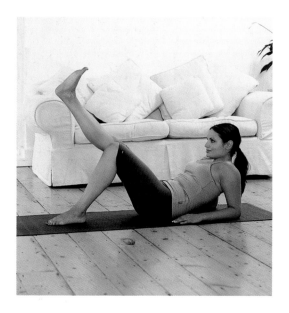

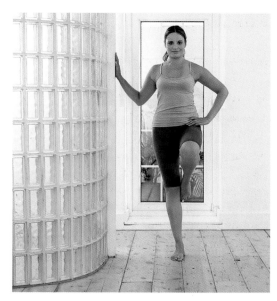

2 KNEE SQUEEZE

✳ Lie on your back on the floor with your arms propping up your upper body behind you. Keep your forearms flat on the floor.

✳ Place your feet flat on the floor and squeeze your bent knees together.

✳ Now simply extend one leg straight and bend it again. Keep your knees pressed together.

✳ Perform three sets of 10 repetitions on each leg.

TRAINING TIP

Vary the exercise by sometimes flexing the foot of the leg you are lifting, sometimes pointing the toe.

---

3 BALLET BARRE LIFT

✳ Stand with your hand against a wall. Bend the outside knee and lift the leg, bringing the foot to touch the supporting knee. Your knee should be pointing forward and your abdominals should be tight, with your back straight and upper body lifted.

✳ Without leaning backwards, extend the bent leg in front of you so that it is straight. The leg should be parallel with the floor and your toes should be pointed.

✳ Hold this position for a few seconds and then bend the leg back in, so that the foot, once again, is tucked in near to the knee.

✳ Perform eight extensions on one leg and then turn around, place your other hand on the wall and repeat on the other side.

4 BALLET JUMPS

Jumping is one of the best ways to tone your thighs – just look at all the sportsmen and dancers on television with fabulous thighs! To jump effectively, however, you need to learn to land correctly.

When landing from a jump, always roll through your feet, then bend your knees. This means letting your toes, followed by the ball of your foot, share the impact with the arch and finally the heel of your foot. When you land from a jump, always press your heels down to the floor with each landing. Never jump and land just on your toes as this puts the Achilles tendon under a lot of pressure and can cause injury.

✳ Stand with your feet slightly apart. Bend your knees and jump into the air, just high enough to stretch your feet and point your toes fully.

✳ Keep your bottom tucked in and abs tight.

✳ Land by rolling through the feet and bending the knees, ready to propel yourself into the next jump again.

✳ Perform 10 jumps in quick succession, then recover and repeat.

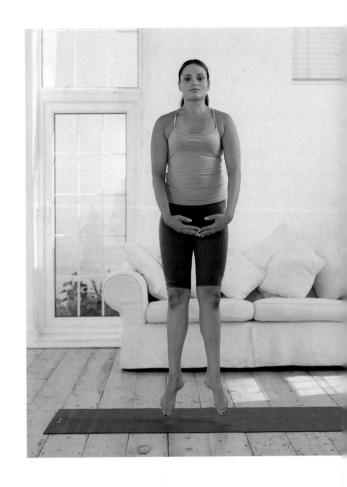

TRAINING TIP
Keep your upper body lifted high with your back straight. Keep your chin up and adopt the perfect posture of a ballet dancer for this exercise.

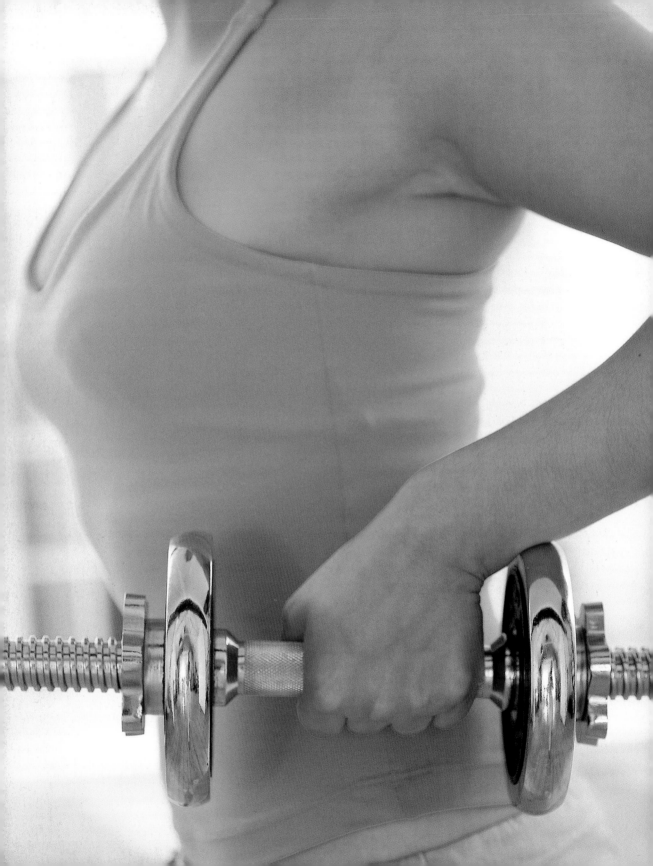

chapter 7

weight training and kick-boxing

Working with weights is key to developing all-round strength and weights are essential tools to aid muscle acquisition. However, weight training does not necessarily mean lifting heavy dumbbells and building bulky muscles to look like a body builder. Rather it involves toning the fibres of the muscles to make them stronger, and defining the shape of the muscle, not enlarging it. Well-toned muscles provide a better body alignment and reduce the appearance of cellulite.

Weight training myths

Weight training is a great way to target and build up muscles in a particular part of your body. Moving your muscles against weighted resistance puts them under stress. As a result, they build in tone and strength. However, there are many misconceptions about what weight training can do.

Training with weights will build muscles but not bulk them up. Don't be afraid of weight training. Unless you lift extremely heavy weights and eat a specialised diet, it is very difficult to bulk up. What does happen is that your muscles will strain slightly and repair themselves, making them more fibrous. This gives the appearance of greater tone as well as increasing strength and giving you a more sculpted appearance. Strengthening your muscles is one of only two ways to change your body shape. The other way is to lose body fat.

You have probably heard it said that muscle can turn into fat and fat into muscle. This is simply not true. They are two separate things. If you train hard you will gain muscle mass and most likely lose body fat. However, if you stop training you will lose muscular tone as it wastes away from lack of use. Without your muscles to raise your metabolic rate and burn calories, you are more than likely to gain some body fat.

Using dumbbells to sculpt your figure

If you are considering purchasing dumbbells to use in your home workout, it is best to use ones that allow you to add or take off weight plates at each end. This ensures that you won't work with one weight for your whole body. Different muscles have different strengths so you may need a range of weights for each exercise.

The biceps, for example, are a set of muscles that get quite a workout over the course of normal activities during your day. These are the arm muscles, used whenever you pick up a shopping bag or reach out and pull something in towards you. They tend, therefore, to remain fairly toned in many people.

To work your biceps effectively, you need to use a weight that is heavier than one you might use for your tricep muscles, which are generally not as strong. Similarly, you might want to use a different weight to work your shoulders than you would to work your back.

Choosing the size of the weight is a matter of practice. You may need to use a relatively heavy weight for some exercises to ensure a good, tough workout. Choose a weight that means that after 12 repetitions you can barely lift it another time. If you can run through 20 repetitions without breaking a sweat then the weight you are lifting is too light for toning your muscles. Increase the size of the weight until you are struggling to achieve 12 repetitions. When you are working at this level regularly, you will see changes in your body shape.

Boosting your biceps

Toning your arms is a goal that can be achieved quite easily. All you need to do is target your arms each week and spend some time completing effective exercises.

For these moves you should use weights. You will see the best and quickest results if you use dumbbells. During the basic bicep curl (opposite) and the preacher curl (page 120), use a weight that tires your biceps after 10 or 12 repetitions. If these exercises seem too easy with a certain weight – that is you could carry on and complete more than 12 repetitions without working hard – increase the size of your weights.

1 BASIC BICEP CURL

✳ Stand tall with your feet hip-width apart and weights in hands by your sides. Bend your elbows, lifting the weights up towards your upper body, with your elbows in at your waist. Slowly lower the weights back down again.

✳ Do a set of 12 repetitions. Make sure you push yourself so that you can hardly lift your arms around the twelfth repetition. Recover and then repeat.

✳ Stretch out your arms after this exercise. Extend your arms out to the side and flex your wrists. Turn your fingertips up to the ceiling and press your arms back behind you a little. You should feel the stretch across your biceps.

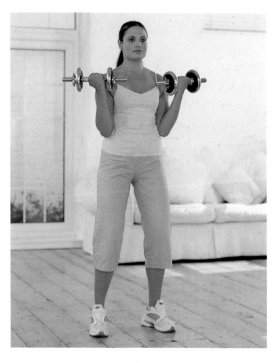

TRAINING TIP
When lifting weights, lowering the weight is equally important as lifting it. Don't be tempted to rush this part. Gravity is on your side but don't allow your arms to fall down quickly. Resisting the pull of gravity on the weight also strengthens the muscle.

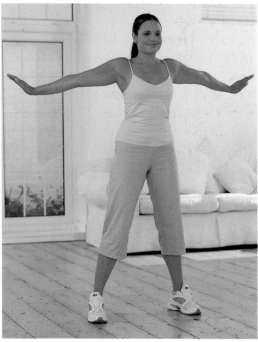

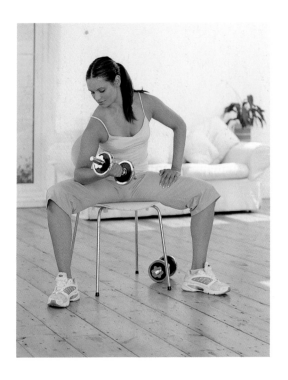

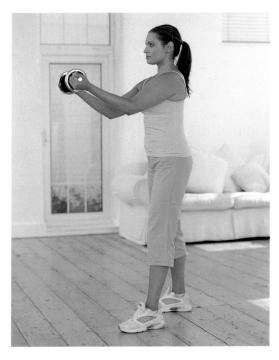

2 PREACHER CURL

✳ Sit on a chair with your legs wide apart. Take one weight in your right hand and press your right elbow against your right thigh. Support yourself with your left hand on your left thigh. While looking at and focusing on the bicep muscles in your right arm, squeeze the muscle to bend the arm to lift and slowly lower the weight.

✳ Perform 12 repetitions, recover and repeat. Repeat the sets of 12 with your left arm.

3 SUSPENDED BICEP CURL

This move works the biceps muscle group at the front of the upper arm as well as the muscles of the shoulders.

✳ Stand with your feet hip-width apart. Hold weights in both hands. Keeping your arms straight, slowly lift your arms so that they are parallel with the floor, facing your wrists towards the ceiling. Keep your stomach tight to support the torso and hold.

✳ Now slowly bend both arms, bringing the weights in towards your body. Slowly extend your arms again and then lower them. Repeat 12 times.

Tricep trials

Many people become concerned about the appearance of the underside of their upper arms. Unlike
the bicep muscles, the triceps do not naturally
remain toned and strong, so they need some
specialised work. As we age, these muscles can
become lax and fat tends to deposit in this region.

    The tricep muscles are stressed by extending
the arm against force. The following three exercises –
tricep dips, tricep extensions, and tricep push-ups –
focus on stretching and stressing these muscles.

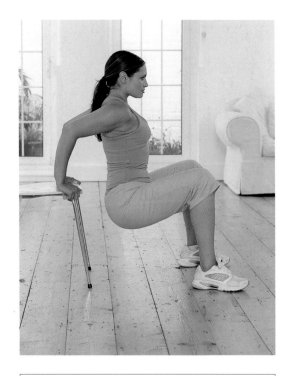

1 TRICEP DIPS

✳ Sit on the edge of a sturdy chair with your
hands on the edge. Walk your feet forward so that
you take your weight on to your feet and hands and
so that your thighs are parallel with the ground.
Keep your upper body straight.

✳ Slowly bend your arms so that your bottom
sinks towards the floor, while your feet remain flat
on the ground.

✳ Straighten your arms to come back to your
original position, lifting your bottom away from
the floor.

✳ Perform 15 to 20 repetitions. Recover and
repeat.

TRAINING TIP
As you straighten your arms and lift your
body back up to its starting position, try
not to push with your legs to bring you up.
This removes much of the stress and work
from the triceps and renders the exercise
virtually ineffective.

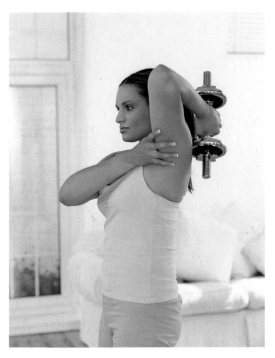

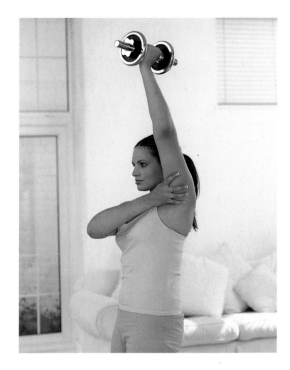

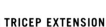

TRICEP EXTENSION

✳ Stand tall with your feet hip-width apart and left hand gripping a weight by placing your left forefinger and thumb around the bottom neck of the weight.

✳ Lift your arm up straight and above your head. Use your right hand to support your left, checking the weight-bearing arm does not slip forward.

✳ Slowly bend your left elbow, tipping the weight behind you, over your shoulder. Hold this position while you check your posture. Keep your abdominal muscles tight and pull in your coccyx.

✳ Extend your arm again, pushing the weight up towards the ceiling. When your arm is straight,

slowly and carefully lower the weight down behind your shoulder again.

✳ Perform 15 repetitions on each arm.

TRAINING TIP
Use your supporting arm to make sure your weight-bearing arm is adopting the correct posture. Be careful to check the weight-bearing arm doesn't slip forwards or backwards in an uncontrolled matter. Take it slowly and you will avoid strains or injuries.

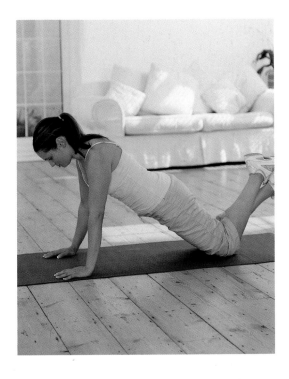
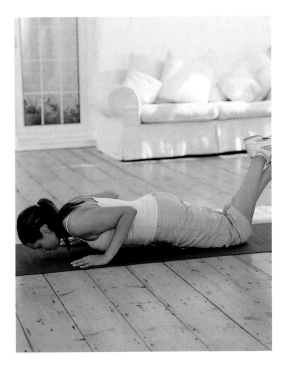

3 TRICEP PUSH-UPS

✱ Kneel on all fours, keeping your back straight. Walk your knees behind you two steps and press your hips all the way forward until your body is in a straight line with much of your weight on your hands.

✱ Move your elbows into your sides, so that they are against your ribcage.

✱ Bend your arms and lower your body slowly towards the floor, keeping your elbows tucked tight into your sides. Your body should be in a straight line – don't allow it to sag in the middle – with your nose and stomach equal distance (approximately 2 centimetres) from the floor. Complete 20 repetitions, recover and repeat.

TRAINING TIPS

Make sure you keeping your elbows in close to your sides when performing this exercise. This is the way to ensure that the move isolates and targets the triceps.

This movement targets the back of the arms. The tough phase in the tricep push-up is pushing your arms straight. If you can't manage 20 repetitions, attempt as many of these push-ups as you can, being careful to keep the correct technique. Never compromise on technique in order to get through more repetitions of a particular exercise.

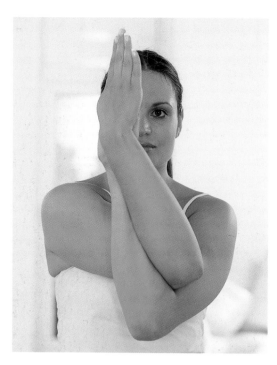

Yoga arms

These yoga moves help to stretch and mobilise the arms. Include them in your home workout when you need to loosen up a little. Performing these exercises will improve circulation to the arms and ease stiffness in the shoulders and arm joints.

1 EAGLE ARMS

✳ Stand tall (or if your yoga is getting good, stand on one leg).

✳ Breathe in as you extend both arms out to the side. Now cross them in front of you with your right arm over your left. Bring your forearms up in front of you with your fingertips pointing upwards.

✳ If you can, try to press both of the palms of your hands together and hold while you move the elbows round in a circle, first one direction then the other. This may feel like quite a stretch when you start, so only do what feels comfortable. If you can't get your palms together initially then just press your arms together. As you continue to practise, your mobility will develop.

2 REVERSE PRAYER

✳ Stand tall and bring both arms behind your back. Press your palms together, with your fingers pointing upwards towards your head and try to press your fingertips together.

✳ Press your hands together and hold for five breaths, feeling the stretch along your arms.

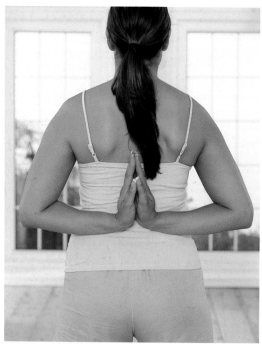

3 INCLINED PLANE

✳ Sit on the floor with your legs straight out in front of you. Place your arms and hands behind you, with your fingertips pointing away from you.

✳ Lean back on your hands and lift your hips high into the air, while dropping your head back. Imagine the whole of the front of your body arching upwards to the ceiling. At the same time, press down through your feet, legs and hands as you hold this position and take two breaths.

✳ Slowly lower yourself back towards the floor and bring your head forward. Repeat this move three times.

4 FOUR-LIMBED STAFF

✳ Kneel on all fours on the floor, with your hands under your shoulders and your knees under your hips.

✳ Tuck your toes under and push your hips up towards the ceiling so that your body forms an upside-down V shape.

✳ Take your weight slightly forward over your shoulders as you bring your hips forward and lower the body into a push-up position.

✳ Hold this position and breathe for five breaths. Use the abdominal muscles and the strength in your arms to hold the position steady. Repeat three times.

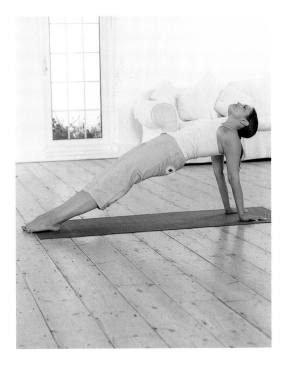

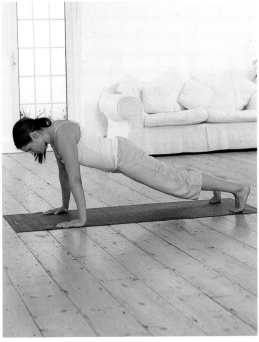

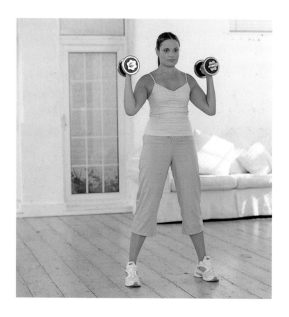

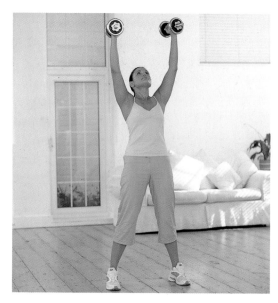

Working your chest and shoulders

The chest and shoulders also benefit greatly from being challenged with weights, so try to include these in your weekly home workout routine.

1 SHOULDER PRESS

✳ Stand tall with your feet hip-width apart and weights in your hands by your sides.

✳ Bend your elbows and lift the weights upwards until the weights are by your shoulders. Your elbows should be positioned out to the sides.

✳ From this position extend your arms up forcefully, lifting the weights up towards the ceiling.

✳ Slowly lower the weights down again to shoulder level. Repeat 18 to 20 times.

TRAINING TIPS

When you straighten your arms, don't slam them completely straight. This can damage your joints. Take care to extend your arms without locking your elbows.

You may feel the deltoid muscles in your shoulder tiring as you perform this exercise. If necessary, rest briefly before resuming the set.

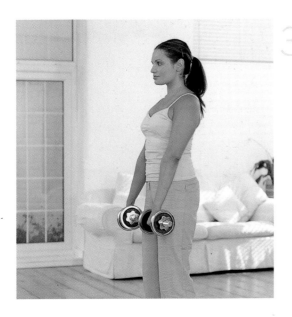

3 PEC DEC

Before you start: for this move you ideally need to lie on a raised surface. If you have a step or bench handy, use this. However, you could use a bed or, failing that, the floor.

✳ Lie on your back with weights in each hand.

✳ Take your arms out to the side, keeping them slightly bent, with your palms facing upwards.

✳ Slowly bring the knuckles of your two hands towards each other. Stop when your hands are 1 centimetre apart.

✳ Open out your arms and bring them back down towards the floor. If you are on a raised surface you can lower the elbows just below the line of your body so that the lift upwards is a little more challenging. Repeat 20 times.

2 DELTOID RAISE

✳ Stand tall, with your stomach tight and shoulders back. Position your feet hip-width apart and hold weights in both hands in front of your thighs.

✳ Raise both arms straight out in front of you until the weights are level with your chest.

✳ Hold for a second and then slowly lower the arms down again.

✳ Perform 20 repetitions of this exercise, then rest for 20 seconds.

```
TRAINING TIP
Vary this exercise by taking your arms out
to your sides when you lift the weights.
```

Boxing arms

Boxing is a great way to combine cardiovascular exercise with an arm-toning workout. And kick-boxing has taken off as a popular cardio sport in cities all around the world. The beauty of kick-boxing is that anyone can do it and it's a superb way to unwind at the end of a hard day and release any pent-up aggression or frustration. Shadow boxing is a technique where you don't hit anything, but practise on an imaginary opponent.

Clear a space in your designated workout area where you can move around a little and swing your arms without hitting anything precious. Gear yourself up to bop around and punch with vigour and intent. Stay on your toes and don't forget your posture. Keep your ribcage lifted and your abdominals tight. Keep breathing regularly as you punch and shuffle.

1 THE 'ALI' SHUFFLE

✳ Lift up your hands and curl them into fists. Tuck the thumbs over the fingers and raise your fist near to your chin. This is where boxers keep them to protect their face.

✳ Bounce from one foot to another in skipping fashion. Keep this jigging constant as you run through the arm moves.

2 THE JAB

✳ With your left fist starting up by your face, shoot your right arm out directly in front of you, palm to the floor, and then recoil it back into the body immediately.

✳ Now bring your arm straight back to shield your face again.

✳ Perform five jabs with your right arm, stepping forward with your right leg as you punch. Bounce back to two feet in between each punch. Repeat with your left arm.

TRAINING TIPS

When you extend your arm, shoot it out as if you are trying to hit someone hard on the jaw. You have to call upon real aggression to get the most out of these moves. Think of someone you'd like to punch, then vent your frustrations through exercise rather than in real life!

Don't get into the habit of slamming your arms so straight that you feel pain in your elbow joints. Shoot your punching arm straight with vigour but don't overextend the elbow joint.

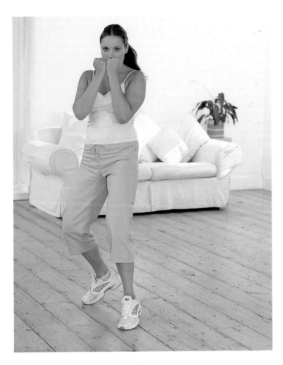

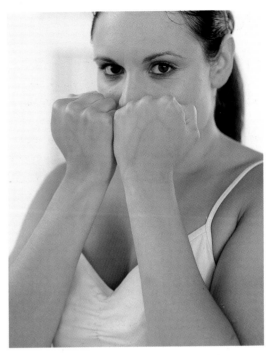

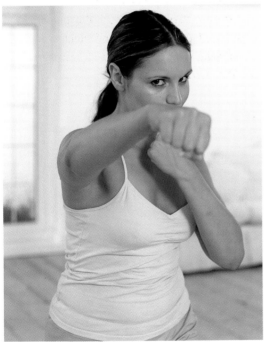

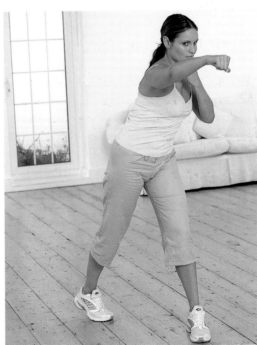

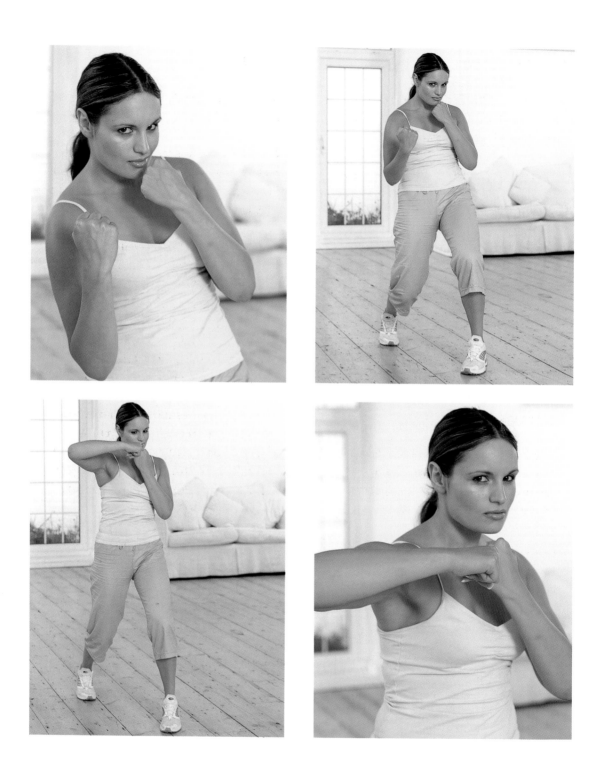

3 THE UPPERCUT

✳ The swing of the arm for this move starts in your legs. Bend both your legs and swing your fist from down beside your body upwards.

✳ Use your whole body to swing into this move by pushing up on your toes on the same side as you swing.

✳ Swing and punch upwards with each arm eight times on each side. Bounce on your toes in between to recover.

TRAINING TIPS

You are aiming to hit your imaginary opponent underneath their jaw in this move. Put your whole body into each punch to gain force.

Use your foot to pivot your whole body into the move. This is how boxers get their knock-outs! They put their whole body weight behind the power of each punch.

---

4 THE HOOK

✳ Lift your leading elbow so that your arm is parallel with the floor.

✳ Push off your toes to swing your arm with the whole weight of your body behind it into a side punch. You are aiming to swing a punch at the side of your imaginary opponent's head.

✳ Keep your arm lifted and your elbow bent and perform eight hooks with each arm. Bounce on your toes in between to recover.

TRAINING TIPS

Turn your whole body to increase the impact of the punch.

Once you have learned these three moves you can intersperse them with your 'Ali' shuffle. You can start to combine the moves in different combinations and perform your own boxing cardiovascular routine, toning your arms at the same time.

Keep shuffling and punching and you will notice yourself breathing harder. The more shuffling and bouncing you do, the more you work your cardiovascular system as well as your arm and leg muscle groups.

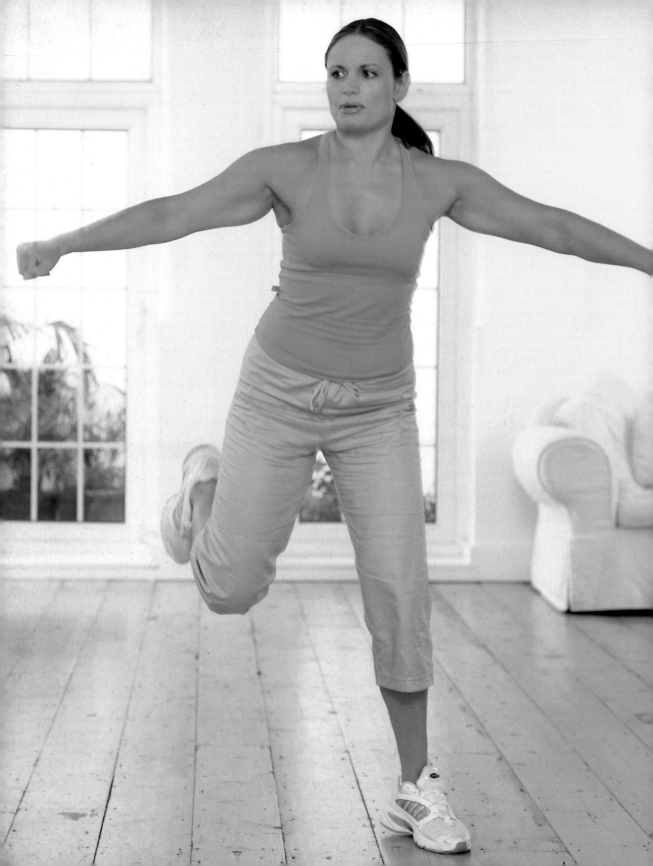

chapter 8

sequence and circuit training

Endurance is about being able to keep going when the going gets tough. It is not until you are out of your comfort zone that you call upon your levels of endurance to find extra energy. Sequence and circuit training push the body to find those extra energy stores. A workout routine where you combine high-intensity moves with low-intensity exercises in order to push your limits is a fun way to achieve this.

Sun salutation sequence

The discipline of yoga has been used to promote endurance and strength for centuries. Start with this well-known routine to help build stamina. Your goal is to build up to being able to perform it 20 times in a row. This takes some doing and it may be a few months before you can manage it – but keep trying because you will notice a world of difference in your levels of endurance and flexibility if you do so.

Many yoga gurus use this sequence before they begin the main yoga practice. As the weeks go by, if you can fit in a Sun Salutation practice every other day you will begin to notice a significant increase in your core body strength. If you need proof, step into a handstand and you will find your point of balance. This is because you have realigned your body and built your endurance and stamina to support it.

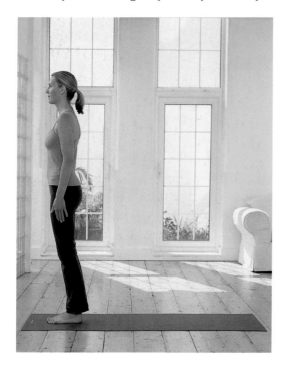

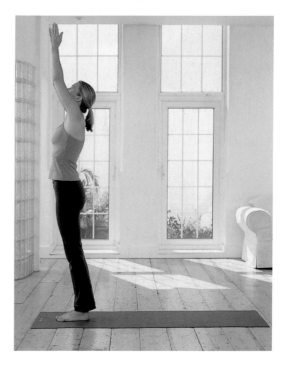

✱ Stand very straight with your legs and feet together, thighs and pelvic floor muscles tight and abdominals firm. With your arms by your sides, lift your body up tall through your ribcage all the way to the top of your head. Check your weight is spread between the balls, heels and big toes of your feet and that it is evenly balanced.

✱ Reach both hands out straight to your sides and then lift them slowly above your head.

✱ Lean your upper body back slightly and tilt your head until you are gazing towards your hands.

✱ Press your palms together and breathe in.

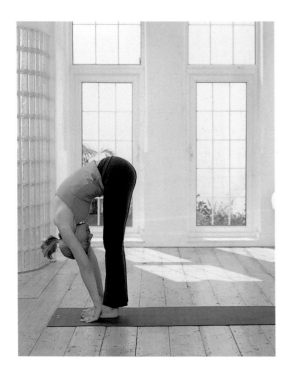

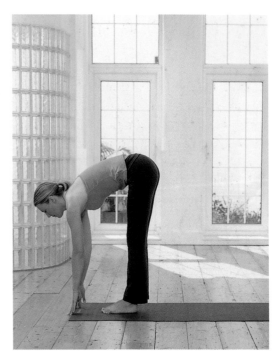

✻ Breathe out as you curve your upper body downwards over your legs to place your hands on the floor in front of your feet. Your arms should be straight. Your head should now be pressing in towards your knees. If you can't quite get this position, don't worry. Simply bend your knees and do your best. As you repeat this sequence as part of your weekly routine, you'll surprise yourself with how much you improve in flexibility in this position.

✻ Breathe in, keeping your hands down on the floor. Slowly begin to straighten your spine, lifting your head away from your knees and keeping your arms straight and pointed towards the floor.

✻ Bend your knees and move your weight to your hands rather than feet. Keep your hands a little wider than hip-width apart.

> TRAINING TIP
> One of the purposes of yoga postures is to build up heat in the body. The body then becomes warm, more pliable and able to perform strength moves more easily.

> TRAINING TIP
> As you move through the sequence you will start to notice a rhythm and flow from one posture to the next. Keep moving through the postures as though it were a slow, controlled dance.

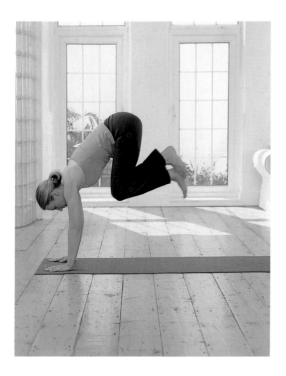 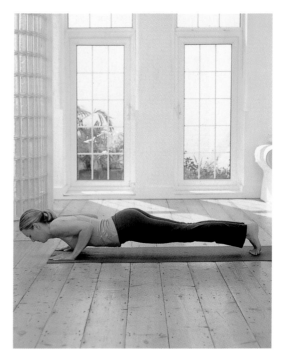

✳ Carefully jump both feet back into a push-up position. If you don't feel that you can jump both feet back in one manouevre (this will come with practice), simply step one foot back first and then the other until you are in a push-up position. If you can jump back but find this move puts pressure on your back or feels excessively uncomfortable, practise first with the step back method until you build sufficient strength to be able to perform the move safely.

✳ Press down through your arms, straighten them, and push your hips forward.

TRAINING TIP

When you first learn the Sun Salutation sequence it can seem confusing and hard to remember. But stick with the practice and your body will soon memorise the movements. Soon you will be able to concentrate less on remembering the moves and more on your breath, gaze and calming your thoughts.

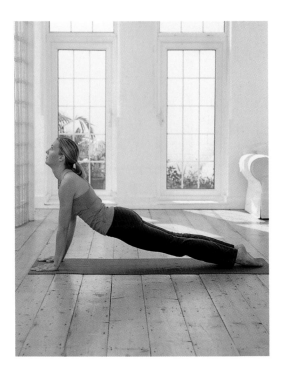

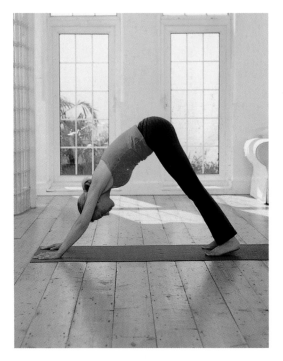

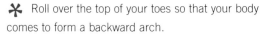

✱ Roll over the top of your toes so that your body comes to form a backward arch.

✱ If you can manage it, keep your hips just off the floor and hold your legs tight and straight.

✱ Open your chest, press your shoulders back and breathe in deeply.

TRAINING TIP

Try to keep the movement from one posture to the next as smooth and calm as possible. Keep in mind that the Sun Salutation is both a physical exercise and a meditation for the mind.

✱ Breathe out as you lift your hips and bottom high into the air. Use your abdominal muscles to achieve this. Press your heels towards the ground. This is the downward dog pose (see page 53). Your body should form an upside-down V shape, with your legs, arms and back staying very straight. This position involves a struggle of forces. While you press back on your heels, you should also be trying to press the front of your thighs towards your stomach, and your armpits towards the floor, as you extend your arms. If you can't perform this move straight away, don't worry about it. You will build up to it as your fitness increases and come to find this position a fabulous stretch across several of the main muscle groups.

✱ Remain in this position for five breaths, giving you time to settle into the position.

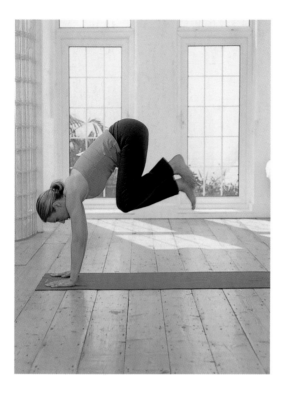

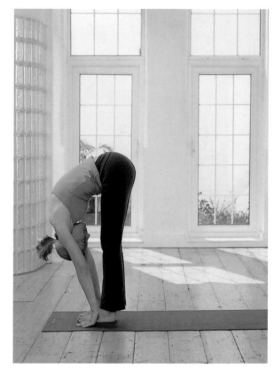

✳ Now prepare to push off with both feet. In the beginning, you may need to rock a little on your toes to ready your body to jump back again.

✳ Push off with your feet and aim to lift your bottom high in the air. Shift all of your weight onto your hands, as if you were about to perform a handstand. Keep your legs bent.

✳ Land your feet between your hands.

✳ Extend your upper body, keeping your hands on the floor and legs straight. Breathe in.

✳ Bend down, folding your upper body back in towards your legs.

✳ Press your head into your knees, keeping your legs straight and breathe out.

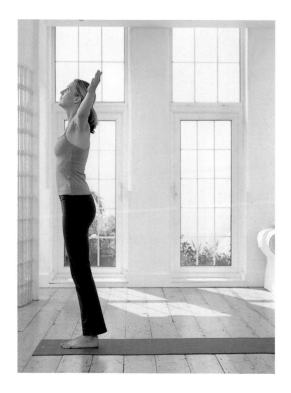

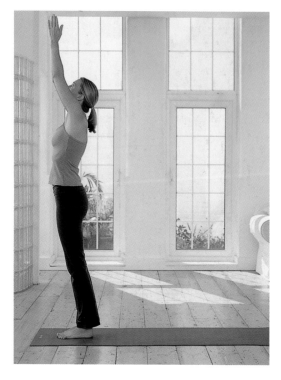

✱ From this folded-up position, breathe in, slowly uncurl your back and lift your arms out straight to the sides.

✱ Reach both palms up and press them together above your head. Keep your arms very straight, just as you did at the beginning of the sequence.

✱ Look up to your thumbs and stretch up straight throughout your whole body.

✱ Lower your arms to the sides of your body and, keeping tall, breathe out.

The sequence is now complete and you are ready to begin again from the start.

Express circuit

Here is an endurance workout based around the circuit principle. Unless you have a very large indoor space, this circuit is probably best done out of doors, in a garden, park or other green patch.

This circuit is designed to push your oxygen intake and build your heart and lung capacity. Jolt yourself out of your comfort zone with a fast and furious six-station circuit. If you complete this entire workout once, allowing for a five-minute warm-up (see chapter 3) and five-minute cool-down (see chapter 9), it should take you 22–25 minutes.

Start by establishing the workstations for your circuit. There will be six stations with different exercises to go to, and between each station you should allow yourself only one minute to rest. Work out at each station for one minute.

The 'resting minute' isn't perhaps quite what you would expect. During each 'rest minute', skip lightly from one foot to the other while you recover your breath. No sitting down and relaxing here!

STATION 1: SPRINT

✳ Pick a distance of about 100 metres. Sprint the distance, forward and back again, for the full minute.

STATION 2: STAR JUMPS

✳ Start by standing tall, with your feet together and your hands loosely by your sides.

✳ Jump and land with your feet wide apart and arms stretched out above your head, roughly forming a star shape.

✳ As you land, bend the knees and then rebound into the next star jump.

> ### TRAINING TIPS
> Keep the pace of the star jumps fast. The moves should be bouncy rather than jerky.
>
> Don't forget to keep breathing deeply as you work out at these stations.

STATION 3: BALLET JUMPS

✳ Stand with your feet together and your toes very slightly turned out, with arms by your sides.

✳ Bend your knees and spring off both feet so that you jump into the air and can point the toes of both feet underneath you.

✳ As you land, make sure you roll through the feet – through the toes, balls of your feet and finally heels. Bend your knees as you land.

✳ From this bend you will have the power to spring upwards into the next jump again.

STATION 4: KNEE JACKS

✳ Position yourself on your hands and knees with your bottom slightly raised in the air.

✳ Lift yourself up on to your toes.

✳ Bring one knee up towards your chin and then quickly swap your legs to bring the other knee up to a similar position.

✳ Swap your legs back and forth as fast as you can for the full minute.

STATION 5: SQUAT THRUSTS

✳ Position your body as you did for station 4.

✳ Push off your feet to jump both knees in under your chest and then thrust both legs out again to land in a push-up position.

✳ Perform as many of these squat thrusts as you can in the minute available.

STATION 6: JOGGING ON THE SPOT

✳ Start on your toes, lift your knees, pump your arms and jog as fast as you possibly can.

✳ Move your feet and arms quicker than you would if you were jogging down the street, so that your limbs are pumping as fast as they can in the time provided.

TRAINING TIP

Don't forget to place a bottle of water somewhere handy. While you take your minute break, have a few sips of water. Particularly during a strenuous workout, it's important to drink plenty of liquids. A hydrated body performs better and recovers quicker.

Power circuit

This circuit focuses on building muscular strength and power. You will feel the effort more in your muscles than in your heart and lungs.

There are only four stations in this circuit. Aim to work out at each station for one and a half minutes. The moves in this workout are high-energy and high-impact, so be careful that you get the technique spot on as you carry out each exercise, otherwise you could cause injury. You will need to pace yourself so that you can keep going for the full one and a half minutes.

This is a 30-minute workout, with a rest period of one minute between stations. Don't forget to stretch out at the end.

In this circuit, you will need to take a minute to rest between stations in order for your muscles to recover. But don't sit down in the middle of a work-out. Step gently from side to side, shaking out your arms and legs or even holding the odd stretch if it feels good.

TRAINING TIP

If you feel the burning sensation of lactic acid, this means that your muscles are running out of energy. You may need to stop or slow down a little to let your muscles recover. The good news is the stronger you get, the longer it will take for your muscles to run out of power.

STATION 1: WIDE JUMPS

✳ Stand with your feet wide apart and your arms straight out to the sides, parallel with the floor.

✳ Bend your knees and jump up. As you do, bring your legs together and move both hands to touching above your head while you are in the air.

✳ As you land, open your arms and legs out again. Bend your knees and lower your arms to be parallel with the floor once again, just like the starting position.

✳ Try to keep the rhythm of the jumps going so that the landing of one takes you into the lift-off of the next.

STATION 2: STAR SPRINGS

✳ Stand with your feet together and your arms by your sides.

✳ Spring off your feet and shoot your arms upwards into a wide V, while you are shooting your legs out to the sides. Your body should form a star shape in the air.

✳ Land with your feet together and arms once again by your sides. Bend your knees and prepare to spring again.

TRAINING TIP

Star springs are a more energetic, high-speed version of star jumps.

STATION 3: BURPEES

✳ Bend down to put your hands on the floor.

✳ Push off your feet to jump both knees out to land in a push-up position, with hands supporting your weight underneath your shoulders.

✳ Jump your legs back in again and prepare to spring into the next Burpee.

TRAINING TIP

Burpees are a great muscle-tester and excellent at building cardiovascular fitness along the way.

STATION 4: HAND-CLAP PUSH-UPS

✳ Position yourself on all fours. Walk your knees back one step and press your hips forward so that you body is in a straight line.

✳ Bend your arms to do a push-up.

✳ From the bent-arm position, push back forcefully with your arms to propel your hands off the floor.

✳ Clap your hands together in the air before taking your weight back on to them.

✳ Bend your arms to absorb the impact ready for the next push-up.

Boxing circuit

Use the boxing ring to provide inspiration for this endurance workout. Most boxers go into the ring for 12 to 15 three-minute rounds. You won't have to complete quite so many rounds with this workout. (Let's pretend you knock out your opponent in the tenth!) Give it a try to push those muscles.

Start with a warm-up and then go straight into a three-minute round. Stay on your feet but rest for one minute before your next bout. Ideally, use a watch with a countdown facility on it for this circuit. Set your watch to sound an alarm at the end of each three-minute countdown – that way you won't need to keep looking at your watch when you should be watching your imaginary opponent!

ROUND 1
✳ Start easy and simply bounce on your feet from side to side. Keep moving and dancing. This is the 'Ali' shuffle (see also page 128).

ROUND 2
✳ Keep moving from side to side but start to practise your jabs (see page 128). Throw a left, throw a right and keep bouncing.

ROUND 3
✳ Start to duck and dive a little. Pretend you have an opponent who is throwing some punches at your head, so you need to duck down low to avoid them. Use your legs and back to bend and then bob back up. Keep shuffling the whole time.

ROUND 4
✳ Try some speed-ball work. Stand upright, bouncing on your toes, and revolve your fists around each other as if you were pummelling a ball, fist over fist. Do this as fast as you can.

ROUND 5
✳ Keep bouncing and add the hook punch (see page 131). Swing your arm around the side and use the twist of your body to really hit hard! Be sure to work out both arms.

ROUND 6
✳ With your legs wide apart, bend one leg and lean to the side. Now bend to the other side. Swing from side to side, punching forwards as you go.

ROUND 7
✳ Stand up on your toes again and dance for a while. Work in some star jumps, with your hands and legs wide. Complete 10, then dance on the spot for a while longer.

ROUND 8
✳ Hit the floor and do some push-ups! Do a set of 10 then leap up and do the 'Ali' shuffle for around 30 seconds. Then hit the floor again.

ROUND 9
✳ Try some imaginary shoe shining. Skip backwards, swinging your feet out to the side and swing your hands, at chest height, over the top of your shoes as if you were giving them a clean.

ROUND 10
✳ Hit the floor and this time lie on your back to perform a fast sit-up set. Curl your head and shoulders in close to your knees and ankles and do some fast pulsing. Try to do 50, then roll over onto your stomach and stretch back.

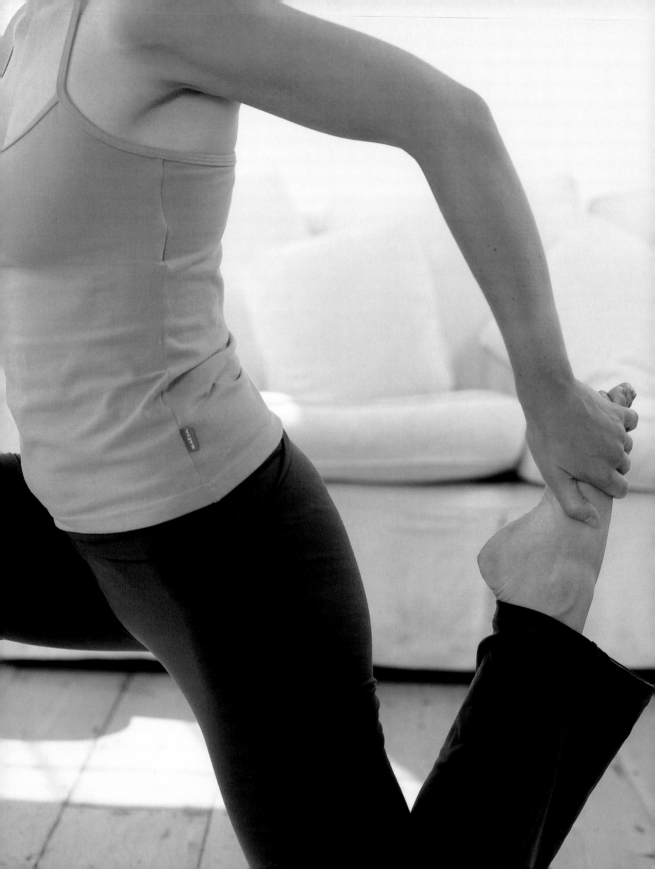

chapter 9

stretching and wind-down

Stretching is a very important part of any fitness routine. Stretching out – that is, lengthening your muscles after exercise – helps return to their original length, reduces the chances of injury and tightness and combats the muscle stiffness that can occur after working hard. A stretching programme can really improve flexibility and mobility, enhancing your ease of movement and posture. Stretching exercises are also a great way to cool down and bring the body and mind into a calm, relaxed state. Don't forget to add a stretching component to each workout you perform.

Stretching theory

There has been some dissent among fitness experts about stretching. Some suggest that stretching is not necessary. They maintain that the body relaxes its muscles of its own accord after exercise. Others suggest that stretching can be harmful if it is performed when the body is cold and can lead to muscles being pulled or torn. It is true that you should take care stretching when you are not warmed up. However, most people in the fitness community acknowledge that stretching is an important part of keeping fit and should be practised regularly.

You can probably draw on your own experience to bear this conclusion out. If you haven't performed a certain move in a while, do you notice that when you come to do it you feel a bit creaky? If you don't extend your limbs regularly, your mobility will lessen. If you don't use your muscles, they will weaken. If you don't continue using movement paths and keep your joints, ligaments and tendons stretched, your body will tighten up.

Keeping a full range of movement is key to feeling ready and able to approach any task. Don't allow movements that were easy to complete as a child to slip away as you age. Keep twisting and bending to maintain the flexibility you enjoyed then.

Coping with muscle stiffness

Stretching after a tough workout may not completely avoid stiffness in your muscles. Stiff, sore muscles are usually the result of overworking your muscles or using muscles that are not used to it. In most cases this occurs a day or two after you've exerted yourself. Scientists believe stiffness may be caused by microscopic tears in the muscles. If you suffer very sore muscles, take a hot shower, try some gentle stretching (as much as you can bear) or even take an aspirin to help you over the discomfort. As you keep exercising you will suffer less from stiffness.

The benefits of stretching

Stretching your muscles back to their original length is very important after you exercise. When you work out you are contracting the muscles rhythmically, repeatedly and with force. After such activity the act of holding the muscles in a stretch, so that they can relax out of the contraction and return back to their original length, gives many of the following benefits:

▶ You will prevent bulky growth of the muscle by encouraging fibres to form over the lengthened belly of each muscle.

▶ You will maintain a full range of movement by keeping your joints mobile.

▶ You will help prevent injuries; a more mobile muscle tears less easily.

▶ You will build strength and flexibility.

▶ You may extend your flexibility and mobility in areas it may be lacking as you complete more challenging stretching routines.

▶ Stretching can reduce the effects of stiffness after intense exercise.

▶ Stretching is a great first step to getting back into fitness if you have been ill or are recovering from an injury.

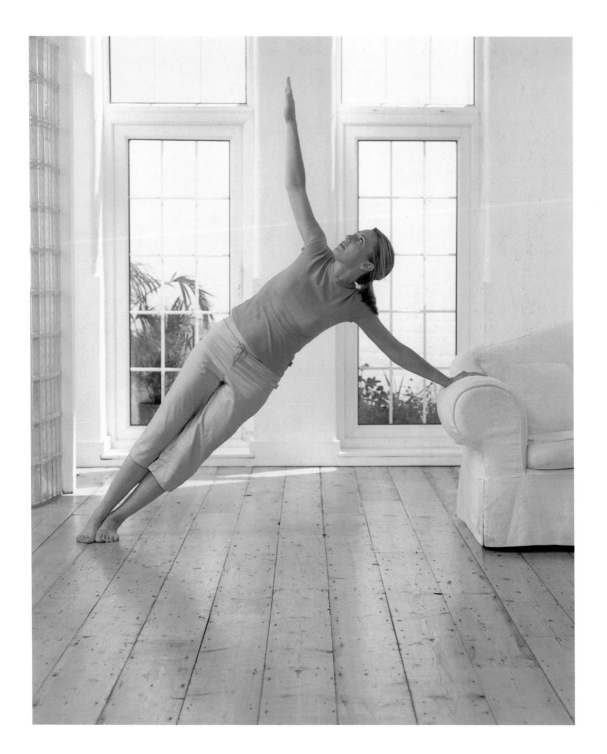

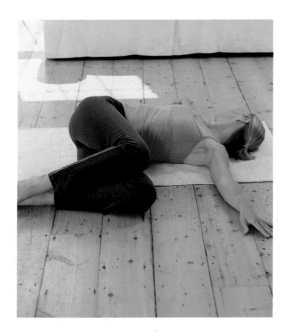

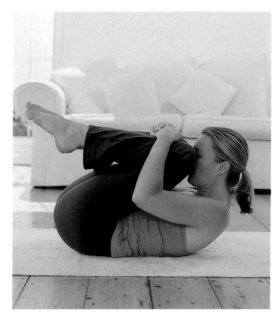

Stretching the spine

The spine is subject to a lot of stress, even from everyday movements such as walking, standing and sitting. The spine is made up of vertebrae with cartilage in between to allow for some movement but it does rely heavily for its health on the body being 'stacked' in the right way and the stomach muscles being toned enough to support it. Stretching the area in and around the spine can help cure muscle tightness that may be causing problems and can help keep the spine flexible and mobile.

1 KNEE TIP

✳ Lie on your back with your feet flat on the floor, knees bent and together. Position your arms flat on the floor, at an angle to your body. Contract your stomach and pelvic floor muscles.

✳ Very gently tip both knees to one side. Tip your knees as far as is comfortable for you – if you can, tip them right the way over until your knees are resting on the floor. Look away from your knees over the opposite hand.

✳ Hold this position for 15 seconds.

✳ Perform this move again, tipping your knees to the other side of your body.

2 KNEE HUG

✳ Lie on the floor and bend both legs up into your chest.

✳ Wrap your arms around your legs, lift your head to meet your knees and breathe in.

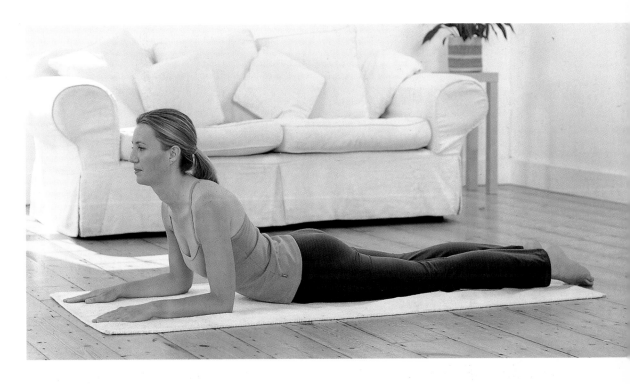

✳ Breathe out and pull your knees tight in to your chest.

✳ Complete this stretch four times taking four deep breaths.

TRAINING TIPS

The knee hug stretches out the lower back and will feel blissful after a hard workout.

Don't forget to stretch out your abdominal muscles as well as your spine after doing any abs work.

---

3 THE SPHINX

✳ Lie on your front and place your elbows and hands on the floor with your back slightly arched.

✳ Relax into this position and press your hips into the floor. This stretches the front abdominal muscles and you may feel some movement in your lower back. If you have no pain in this position you can move on to the next stage.

✳ Press on your hands and lift your elbows off the floor, arching your body further back. Hold this position for 15 seconds and then slowly release.

Stretching the legs

Don't neglect to stretch out your leg muscles. Your legs bear the weight of your body every day. Tight legs can cause back problems and unbalanced leg muscles can cause problems in the knees and ankles. Regular stretching of the large muscles at the front and back of the thigh – the hamstrings and quadriceps – will help to realign the joints and keep them healthy.

1 HAMSTRING STRETCH

✳ Lie on your back on the floor with legs straight.

✳ Bend one knee in towards your chest and hug your knee close to your body. Hold for three seconds.

✳ Hold on to your lower calf and extend your leg up to the ceiling, or if you can, towards your face. Keep your knee bent if necessary. You will feel this stretch all along the back of the leg.

✳ Breathe in, then breathe out and gently try to pull the leg nearer to your face. Repeat with the other leg.

TRAINING TIP
This exercise stretches the hamstring muscle at the back of your thigh. Only pull the leg in until you feel a mild to medium stretch in the back of your leg – stop if you feel any pain.

---

2 QUADRICEPS STRETCH

✳ Lie on your stomach on the floor and bend one leg up behind you towards your buttock.

✳ Raise your upper body, resting on one elbow.

✳ Take your other hand and grasp the foot of your bent leg. Pull your foot gently into the buttock and hold. You will feel a stretch down the front of your thigh.

✳ Hold this pose for 15 seconds and then repeat with the other leg. This stretch can also be performed in a standing position.

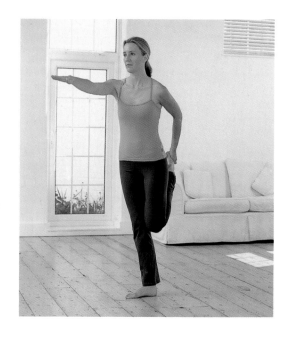

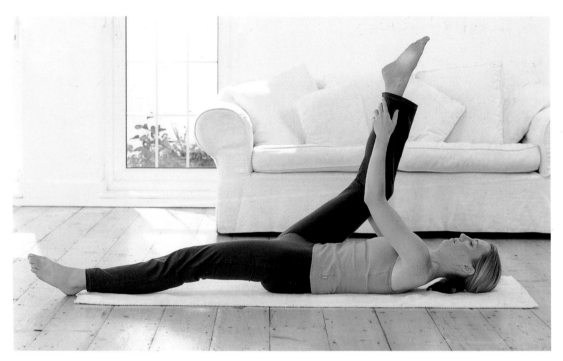

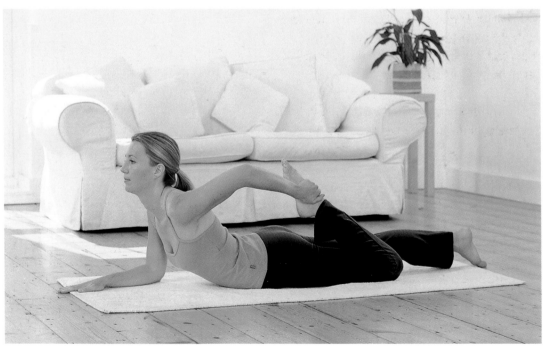

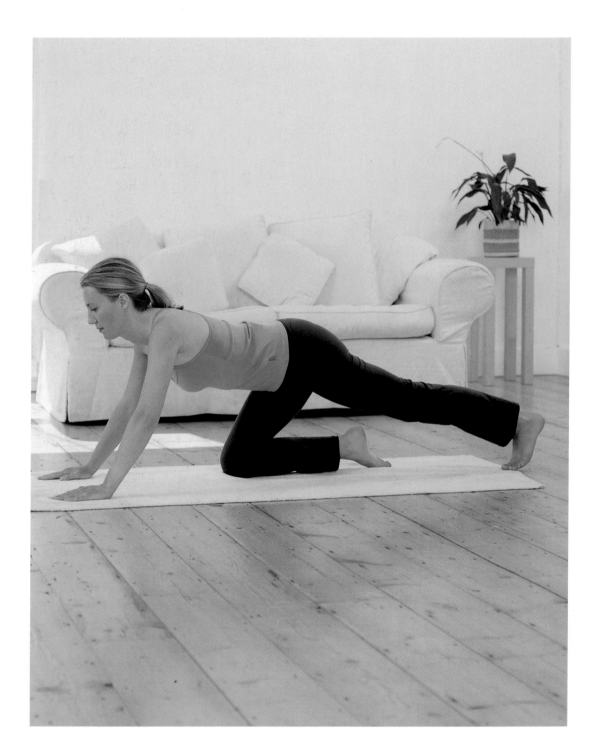

3 KNEELING CALF STRETCH

✻ Position yourself on the floor on your hands and knees. Take one leg straight behind you and use it to anchor yourself onto the floor.

✻ Press the heel of your back leg away from you. You will feel a stretch in your calf muscle.

✻ Hold the stretch for 15 seconds and repeat on the other leg.

4 STANDING CALF STRETCH

✻ Stand with one leg behind the other in a lunge position.

✻ Press the back heel down into the floor as much as you can to feel the stretch at the back of the lower leg. Lean forward slightly to increase the stretch.

✻ Hold the stretch for 15 seconds and repeat on the other leg.

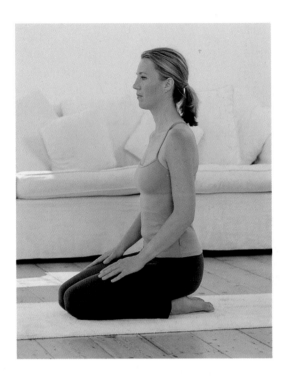

5 TIBIALIS STRETCH

✻ Kneel with your knees together and pointing straight ahead. Place your bottom on your heels. Hold for 10 seconds and relax.

TRAINING TIP

It is very common to get cramps in the calf muscles when cooling down after a strenuous workout. Stretch out these muscles gently to return them to their full length.

TRAINING TIPS

This stretch targets the lower front of the leg and mobilises the knee joints.

Sit in the tibialis stretch position for the full 10 seconds only if it is comfortable.

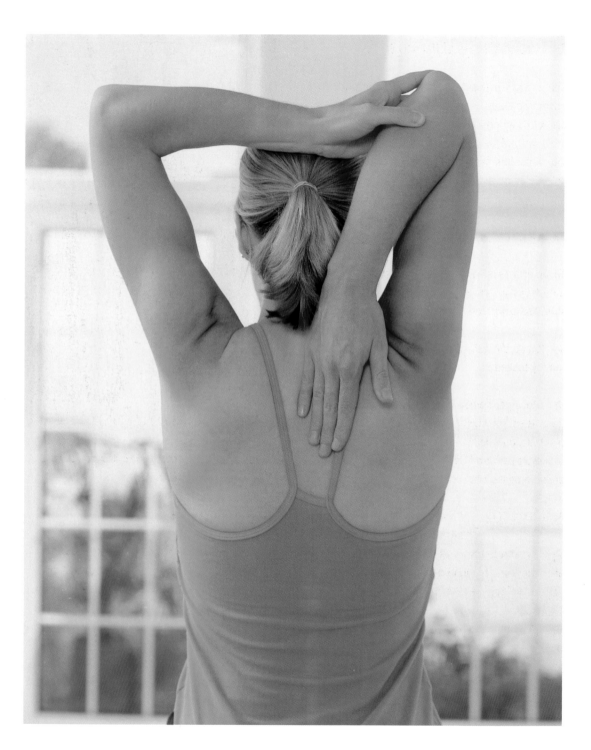

Stretching the arms

Many people overlook stretching the arms and upper body but it is an important area to keep supple. You might have experienced severe stiffness of the arms and shoulders after a tough workout and found that it is painful to drive a car or lift shopping bags. You can avoid this by returning the muscles to their pre-workout length.

1 TRICEP STRETCH

Tricep exercises work the back of the arms and this muscle group can get extremely sore if not stretched out properly.

✱ Stand tall with your feet hip-width apart and tummy tucked in.

✱ Bend your elbow and reach one hand back towards your shoulder blade. With the other hand, pull the elbow back. Keep your upper torso straight while you perform this stretch. Hold for 10–12 seconds. Repeat on the other arm.

2 SIDE STRETCH

✱ Stand with your legs wide apart. Bend one leg and lean towards the bent leg. Make sure the bent knee is directly over the supporting foot.

✱ Reach the arm on the opposite side to the bent leg up straight and then lean your whole body into the stretch. Hold for a few seconds.

✱ Move back from your bent leg and then slowly into the stretch again to make this a moving stretch.

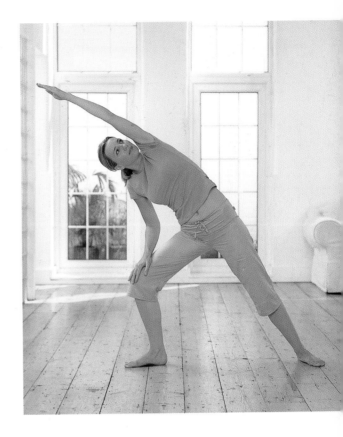

Reach as far as you can with your straight arm. Repeat on the other side.

3 SHOULDER STRETCH

✱ Stand a little away from a wall. Place your hands on the wall and walk your feet away until your upper body is horizontal, with back and arms straight and hands still pressing on the wall.

✱ Press your armpits towards the floor to feel a flexing in the shoulder joints. Press and release a few times to extend the range of movement of the shoulders.

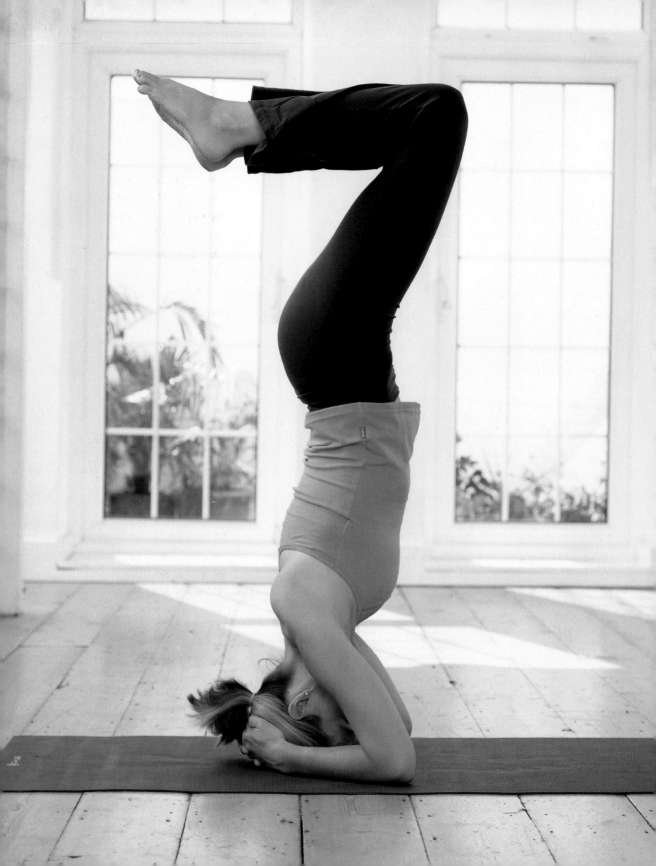

index

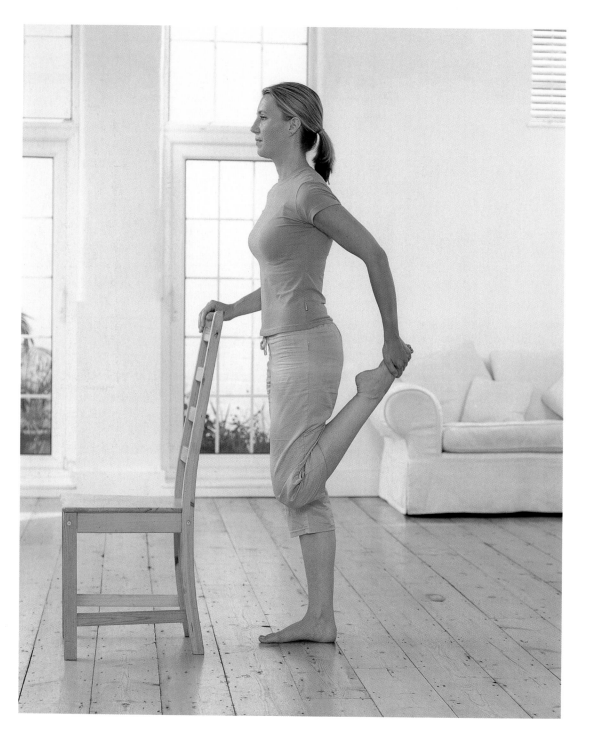